The
PHYSIOLOGY
of
STRESS

WITH SPECIAL REFERENCE TO THE NEUROENDOCRINE SYSTEM

MARY F. ASTERITA, Ph.D.
Indiana University School of Medicine
Gary, IN

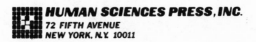
HUMAN SCIENCES PRESS, INC.
72 FIFTH AVENUE
NEW YORK, N.Y. 10011

Printed in the United States of America
987654321

Library of Congress Cataloging in Publication Data

Asterita, Mary F. (Mary Frances)
  The physiology of stress.

  Bibliography: p.
  Includes index.
  1. Stress (Physiology) 2. Neuroendocrinology.
I. Title. [DNLM: 1. Stress—Physiopathology. 2. Stress,
Psychological—Physiopathology. 3. Nervous system—
Physiology. 4. Endocrine glands—Physiology. QT 162.S8
A853p]
QP82.2.S8A85   1985   612   84-6591
ISBN 0-89885-176-9
ISBN 0-89885-187-4 (pbk.)

This book is to be returned on or before
the last date stamped below.

12 DEC 1989
11. DEC 1990
-4 JAN 1991
11. JAN 1993
-3 MAR 1993
17. MAR 1995

2 ᴰ MAR 2010

6th Aug 2013

17 JAN 1998

3 1 OCT 2008

16/4/10

2 8 MAR 2014

Astorita, M.F.

DEDICATED TO

MY FATHER

for upholding the highest principles which guided our lives and for his steadfast devotedness to his family.

MY MOTHER

for her persistent dedication to her family and for guiding her children in the pursuit of the loftiest ideals in life.

MY YOUNGER BROTHER, MARTY,

who by his buoyant spirit has touched the lives of many, and now has left us to journey on to other realms of life.

CONTENTS

PREFACE

In the last decade, the study of stress and the psychophysiology of the stress response itself has gained a prominent place in the whole arena of human health and disease. According to estimates cited on several occasions in the literature, between 75 and 90 percent of all disease prevalent in western society today is related to the activation of the stress mechanism of the body. This fact in itself has created the need to know more about the nature of the stress response, particularly in reference to its physiology. While there are at present several books in print which discuss stress in terms of its nature, relationship to life-style, disease, management, and treatment, there is no book wholly devoted to discussing stress in terms of its physiology.

The main purpose of this book is to present a scientific exposition of the physiology of stress based on general knowledge and current research findings. It is the major emphasis of this text to discuss in general terms the changes resulting in the nervous and endocrine systems of the body, which produce specific end-organ activity as a result of the elicitation of the stress response.

This book is intended to be used as a source book of basic physiology and recent research findings in the area of the Physiology of Stress for practicing clinicians, physicians, psychologists, physical therapists, nurses, and other allied health professionals who frequently encounter clients experiencing illnesses due to an escalated psychophysiological stress arousal state.

The research referenced in this text is related mainly to work which has been reported within the last 30 years, and is by no means inclusive of all the scientific investigations in the field to date. The research work cited has been chosen only for the purpose of being representative of other similar and notable published research. While the text presents only a limited review of the literature, the intent is to give the reader a "feel" for the type of work that is involved in developing and expanding scientific knowledge as it relates to the physiology of the stress response. It is not the intent of this text to present a final definitive work concerning the Physiology of Stress, but to update and bring together key areas of research in this field, particularly with regard to the effects of psychosomatically induced stress on the nervous and endocrine systems.

Mary F. Asterita, Ph.D.

ACKNOWLEDGMENTS

The following individuals deserve much thanks for contributing their time and talents in making this book become a reality: To Dr. Charles Stroebel, Dr. Joel Lubar, and Dr. Edgar Wilson who have reviewed the text and have provided several helpful comments and recommendations; to Ioanna Iatrides, for the initial preparation of the illustrations which appear in Chapters 2, 4, and 6, for initial preparation and organization of the glossary, and for her most valuable technical assistance; to Patricia Healton, for her typing skills in preparing the first draft of this manuscript, for the preparation of the illustrations which appear in Chapters 3, 10, 13, and 16 and for her technical assistance; to Dr. Donald Macchia, for the final preparation of the illustrations which appear in Chapters 2, 3, 4, 5, 6, 10, 13, and 16 and for contributing his professional insight, and his time and efforts in reviewing portions of the manuscript; to Lena Fortier, for contributing much of her time and efforts in typing and applying her word processor skills to this manuscript; to Jean Cifaldi, for her excellent typing skills and for producing this manuscript in its final form; and to all others at the Northwest Center for Medical Education, Indiana University School of Medicine, who contributed their help and professional assistance. I am grateful to those authors and publishers who have granted their permission to reproduce diagrams and figures which have originally appeared in their own publications. Finally, a word of thanks goes to my family and friends for their continuing understanding, encouragement, and loving support.

CHAPTER 1

Introduction

The work of Claude Bernard in the later part of the 19th century focused on the concept that all of life is dependent on precise well-coordinated physiological regulatory mechanisms. Claude Bernard actually saw the importance of viewing the organism in terms of the interactions between all of its bodily processes. He laid the foundation for an integrative approach to the study of the physiology of the organism.

The work of Bernard was followed by the work of several scientists who were concerned with the subject of physiological integration. Among such researchers, was Walter B. Cannon, an eminent physiologist, whose pioneering work of the early 1900's should be noted. Cannon investigated the physiology of the organism from several different points of view. While his focus was primarily on the physiological basis of homeostasis, he also studied the control of the sympathetic nervous system on internal secretions, the influence of the endocrine system on metabolism and the influence of emotional disturbances on various physiological processes. Cannon directed much of his attention to a response which he called the "emergency reaction". He demonstrated that this response can be labelled a "fight or flight" response since its main purpose is to protect the organism and guarantee its survival. When an organism confronts a situation, whether physical, mental, or emotional, which poses as a threat or a danger, then, the choice would be either to face the threat or danger or to flee from it. This "fight or flight" response involves the activation of the sympathetic portion of the autonomic nervous system and the activation of the adrenal medullary axis. This work of Cannon as well as his other scientific investigative work and that of others has led to the establishment of both a theoretical and experimental framework for the field of integrative physiology.

The pioneering investigative work of Cannon was then followed by that of Hans Selye who approached the field of integrative physiology from a psychosomatic point of view. Selye, through his work dealing with the stress response, focused much of his attention on stress-related disorders and the resulting disease states.

The early work of Selye suggested that psychological, that is, both mental and emotional mechanisms appear to play a role in the regulation of the pituitary — adrenal cortical axis. Up to that time, the sympathetic — adrenal medullary axis was the only system known to be responsive to both mental and emotional stimuli. As was mentioned, this was a result of the systematic work of Cannon many years earlier. The pioneering work of Selye and other researchers as well, suggested that other endocrine systems may also come under mental and emotional influences. Today, it is quite evident, that endocrine regulation, in terms of mental and emotional influences, is very likely to be much more broad based, involving multiple endocrine systems or axes in addition to those involving the adrenal medulla and cortex. Continuing scientific investigations by several researchers, dealing with the stress response and stress reactivity within the organism have led to growth and expansion of the field of psychoneuroendocrinology, which is indeed the subject of this text. In addition, to supplement or perhaps even to complement this growing field, the research which investigates the mental and emotional influences on the immune system is leading to the growth and expansion of the new and important field referred to as psychoneuroimmunology.

To summarize, the work of Claude Bernard described integrative physiology in terms of the interrelationships between the various physiological regulatory mechanisms within the organism itself. Now, through the work of various scientists investigating the stress response and stress reactivity, as well as other scientists working in related fields, we are coming to view integrative physiology from a broader perspective. Integrative physiology must be viewed not only in terms of the interrelationships of the physiological regulatory mechanisms which occur within the organism, but must also incorporate the understanding that these mechanisms appear to be influenced by mental and emotional stimuli. This leads directly to a discussion of stress and the stress response since the stress response is associated with physiological changes which occur in the physical body as a result of physical, mental, or emotional influences.

Stress is a common subject of interest. Today it is recognized as a fact of life. The term stress was first described by Selye (1950, 1957). "Stress" pertains to a state produced within an organism subject to a stimulus perceived as a threat (stressor). Selye actually described stress as a common denominator underlying all adaptive responses within the body. He also defined stress ". . . as a state manifested by a specific syndrome which consists of all the nonspecifically induced changes within a biologic system." In other words, the term stress can be used to refer to a wide range of physiological changes induced by various psychological or physical factors (stimuli) or a combination of these factors.

The effect of stress on the body, no matter what the nature, cause, or type of stress involved, results in a specific physiological response by the body and is generally termed the stress response. This stress response is, in reality, a complex response, because it incorporates numerous physiological mechanisms. Stress, to date, has not been precisely defined, but a wealth of scientific knowledge and research data does exist to provide us with a general integrated perspective as to its nature, particularly in physiological terms. Certainly the pioneer work of several scientists, including Selye himself (1976), has contributed much understanding and basic knowledge to the field of stress.

Basic Physiological Concepts

It is known that the organism survives because of the maintenance of a normal internal environment, which is more commonly referred to as homeostasis. Now, any threat (stress) which may occur to disrupt this homeostasis will produce physiological reactions in the body which attempt to resist any such changes taking place. These physiological reactions involve the activity of both the nervous and endocrine systems, which in turn result in various system and end-organ responses. In particular, the outcome of a threat or stress to the organism results in an activation of the autonomic nervous system and a changed endocrine response, with an increase or decrease in secretions of various hormones in the body. It is the aim of this text to focus on the changes occurring in both the nervous and endocrine systems along with their specific physiological effects, as a result of the elicitation of the stress response.

Types of Stress

Any stimuli which an organism perceives as a threat is termed a stressor. Stressors may be physical, psychological, or psychosocial in nature.

Physical stressors include the presence of such conditions as environmental pollutants or other environmental pressures, as for example, extreme changes in temperature. Immobilization and electric shock would be other examples of physical stressors. The concept of a physical stressor may also encompass those stressors which are physiological in nature, such as a decrease in oxygen supply, prolonged exercise, hypoglycemia, injuries, and other trauma to the body.

Psychological stress or psychogenic-induced stress results from reactivity within oneself to one's own personal thoughts and/or feelings about real or imagined threats.

In discussing psychological stress, it is important to emphasize that the mental and/or affective components of human reactivity are included. Psychological stress resulting directly from social interactions is often referred to as psychosocial stress.

Psychosocial stress results from personal responses to intense social interactions, or lack of such interactions, or even perhaps to other subtle social interrelationships. Thus a person may elicit a stress response whether in a state of social isolation or in a state of anxiety about prevailing social interpersonal relationships.

Since the stress response elicited within the body must be viewed from the perspective of the organism as a whole (incorporating both the psychological and physiological (somatic) components), the term psychosomatic stress is often used as well.

It must be emphasized that factors which result in physical, social, and psychological (mental or emotional) stress are different for different people. In other words, what is stressful for one person may or may not be stressful for another person. Here one must also consider temporal variability: that is to say, what may be stressful for one person at a particular time may or may not act as a stressor at a later point.

As stated above, stress to date has not been precisely defined. The term stress is very general and is used quite loosely. There are many ways to describe it. It is not our purpose here to enter into a lengthly discussion of the definition of stress. We all know what stress is since we have experienced it in various degrees at one time or another. We also know what thinking or feeling is because we think and feel all the time. Yet when we come right down to it, we find that it is indeed quite difficult to actually define these concepts. In the same way, it is quite difficult to define stress.

To ease the situation somewhat, Selye spoke of stress in terms of eustress and distress. In this way, stress is described in terms of its positive or negative consequences upon the body. Distress is characterized by an accumulation of negative consequences on the body while eustress is characterized by relatively few. These consequences may become manifest more so in the long term than in the short term.

Another way to describe stress is to state that an organism is stressed when any or some of its constituent parts, whether physical, biochemical, mental, emotional, behavioral, etc. are confronted with a challenge, constraint, or demand (stressor) to do or be at such a level, that a return to baseline does not immediately occur when the stressor is removed. This causes a shift in the homeostasis of the organism. This shift may occur either in the short term or long term. Long term homeostatic changes eventually lead to an alteration or breakdown of any of the constituent parts within the organism. Eustress produces this effect much less than distress does.

With a description of stress in these terms, one must consider the important aspect of perceptivity. The way an individual perceives reality determines the amount, kind, and intensity of stress that will be experienced. The needs, beliefs, and value system of the individual play an important role in determining how the perception of a challenge, constraint, and/or demand will lead to the experience of stress in terms of eustress or distress. Also, the personality characteristics of an individual also play an important role in influencing the perception of the individual as to what constitutes challenge, constraint and/or demand.

So, whatever the stressful condition, factors, or stimuli may be that induce the stress response, the physiological reactions which occur under such conditions are very real, and are the subject of this text.

CHAPTER 2

The Human Nervous System

CELLULAR PHYSIOLOGY

It is of utmost importance for an adequate understanding of the stress response to describe in a general way its neurological basis. Therefore the purpose of this section is to review the basic anatomy and physiology of the human nervous system.

The basic anatomical unit of the nervous system is the neuron (Figure 1). It consists mainly of three parts: the dendrites, the cell body or soma, and axon. Incoming signals are received by the dendrites and transmitted down the axon, away from the cell body, and towards the dendrites of an adjacent neuron or to an end-organ.

The transmission of an electrical signal along a neuron occurs because of simultaneously occurring complex electrical and chemical changes, which result in a changing membrane potential. Under resting conditions, the electrical potential inside the neuronal cell is of the order of -90mV with respect to the outside bathing solution. During the transmission process, this potential changes and becomes less negative. In actual fact, the potential actually reverses

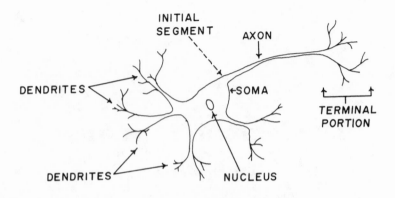

Figure 1
A neuron, the basic functional unit of the human nervous system.

itself, and becomes positive. This is called a depolarization, and this depolarization wave can spread down the axon. Depolarization is often referred to as an action potential and is seen electrically as a change in membrane potential from resting levels, −90mV, to +30 or +40mV. This is a sweeping change in the electrical potential of approximately 135mV. This alteration in electrical potential is accompanied by corresponding changes in the membrane permeability to sodium (Na^+) and potassium (K^+) ions.

Surrounding all cells is the extracellular fluid, which contains large amounts of sodium and chloride, and a small amount of potassium. The reverse is true for the fluids within the cell. During excitation of the cell, it is the sodium and potassium ions that are mainly affected. Cell excitation results in changes in cell membrane permeability to these ions, which allows sodium and potassium ions to flow down their chemical gradients. Since there is more extracellular sodium, this cation will move into the cells, while potassium, for similar reasons, will move out of the cells. The result is that sodium ions will enter the cells while potassium ions

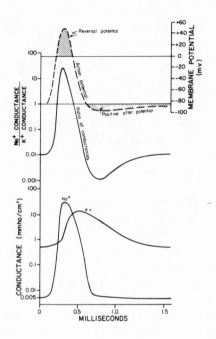

Figure 2

The action potential and the sodium and potassium conductance changes. The upper part of the figure illustrates an intracellular recording of an action potential. Beneath this is shown the parallel changes that take place in the sodium-potassium conductance ratio. The bottom portion of the figure illustrates the individual sodium and potassium conductance changes during the action potential. It can be seen that during the initial portion of the action potential, the conductance of sodium increases several thousandfold, whereas during the action potential, the conductance of potassium increases approximately 30-fold. (Curves constructed from the data in Hodgkin and Huxley papers but transposed from squid axon to apply to the membrane potentials of large mammalian nerve fibers.) Adapted from A.C. Guyton, *Textbook of Medical Physiology*, (6th ed.). Philadelphia: W.D. Saunders Co., 1981, p. 110.

leave the cells. The timing of the membrane permeability changes during excitation and the conductance of each ion across the membranes results in the characteristic action potential — a measurable electrical event (Figure 2). The upper part of Figure 2 illustrates the action potential along with the corresponding changes in the sodium and potassium conductance ratio. The lower part of the figure illustrates the changes which occur in sodium and potassium conductances separately.

The action potential occurs in two separate stages called membrane depolarization, which was discussed above, and membrane repolarization. Almost immediately after depolarization occurs, the membrane closes its channels to sodium ions. Potassium ions then move from inside the nerve cell to the outside. Since the potassium ions are positively charged, the excess positive charges inside the neuron are transferred back out of the cell. The normal negative resting membrane potential is then restored. This aspect of the action potential is called repolarization.

The action potential is of short duration and the whole electrical event, both onset (depolarization) and recovery (repolarization), occurs within the order of milliseconds.

The actual amount of ions transported during the action potential in cell entry and exit is quite small. At the end of each action potential, the active transport of sodium and potassium ions to their original resting levels occurs within a few milliseconds.

Figure 2 depicts the nerve tissue action potential as seen from a recording made with intracellular electrodes. This measurable electrical event forms the basis for such electrophysiological procedures as electroencephalography, electromyography, and electrocardiography. When external electrodes are used, the recording measures biphasic or even triphasic responses depending on the positioning of external electrodes from the site of activity. It must be noted that in a whole muscle or nerve, local current flow is not confined to just the surface of the cell membrane but spreads throughout the tissue due to the presence of an electrolytic solution which surrounds the muscle and nerve fibers. The system as a whole can be viewed in terms of the volume conducting properties of the electrolytic solution surrounding the muscles and nerve fibers. These

VOLUME CONDUCTION AND ELECTROMYOGRAPHY

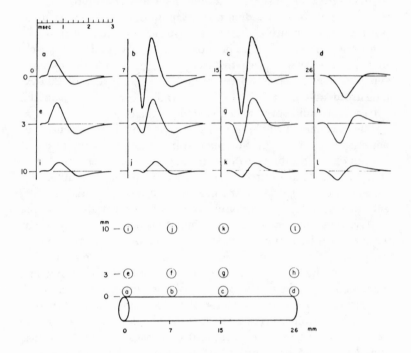

Figure 3

Action potentials recorded with extracellular electrodes. Extracellular potentials recorded at different points along the nerve (a, b, c, d) and at various distances; e, f, g, and h are 3mm from the nerve and i, j, k, and 1 are 10mm. Impulse is initiated from point a. (Adapted from R. Lorente de No, A Study of Nerve Physiology. *Studies from the Rockefeller Institute of Medical Research*, (Vol. 132). New York: The Rockefeller University Press, 1974, p. 466.

recordings although made extracellularly are a reflection of the electrical events occurring at the cellular level. A typical response is seen in Figure 3.

An electrical impulse travels down the neuronal axon to reach its terminal portions, the dendrites. Upon reaching the terminal portions of the neuron, the transmission of an electrical impulse, from one nerve cell to another, or from a nerve cell to a muscle fiber, must cross a space that separates the two cells, called a synapse. The space is relatively small, of the order of 200 A° (angstrom units), or 200×10^{-8}cm and is continuous with the extracellular fluid space which surrounds the cells.

The way in which the impulse is transmitted from neuron to neuron or neuron to end-organ involves changes in the terminal membrane permeability to calcium ions, release of chemical substances (neurotransmitters) across the synapse (presynaptic element) to receptor sites on the next neuron (postsynaptic element) and, finally, changes in sodium and potassium permeabilities of the postsynaptic membrane, resulting in propagation of the impulse or action potential along the postsynaptic neuron. Electrosecretory coupling is the basis of synaptic transmission. Here, the electrical impulse at the terminal portions of the axon of the presynaptic element induces the release of a neurotransmitter substance, which then travels to the receptor sites of the postsynaptic neuron subsequently to excite this neuron. It is the phenomenon of electrosecretory coupling that allows continued propagation of the electrical impulse from neuron to neuron or from neuron to end-organ. There are several endogenous neurotransmitter substances, but those of primary interest in the study of stress are the neurotransmitters of the autonomic nervous system, namely, norepinephrine (noradrenaline) and acetylcholine.

Now, in order for the effect of the neurotransmitter not to persist at the level of the postsynaptic neuron, an enzyme is present which causes the degradation of the neurotransmitter. This is one method of neurotransmitter removal. The activity of acetycholine (ACh) which is the neurotransmitter at certain autonomic neuroeffector sites, and the neuromuscular junction of skeletal muscle, undergoes the process of degradation by the enzyme cholinesterase. This enzyme is located at the membrane of the postsynaptic element.

Another mechanism besides enzymatic degradation to halt neurotransmitter activity and remove it from the synapse, involves sequesterization of the active neurotransmitter. For this purpose a pump is used, not only to transport the specific neurotransmitter out of the synaptic cleft, but to sequester the neurotransmitter back into the interior of the presynaptic terminal. Hence, the neurotransmitter substance is removed from the receptor of the postsynaptic element and is cleared from the synapse. Having entered the terminal portion of the presynaptic element, the neurotransmitter may be broken down by enzymatic activity, or may be taken up by vesicles where it is stored until released again. Examples of neurotransmitters that are removed in this manner include the catecholamines, glutamic acid, glycine, and 5-hydroxytryptamine.

Let us now present a brief discussion of the human nervous system, which is comprised of the central and preipheral nervous systems.

CENTRAL NERVOUS SYSTEM

The brain and the spinal cord form the central nervous system. Anatomically, the human brain is composed of three major parts, namely the cerebrum, the cerebellum, and the brainstem.

The cerebrum is composed of two lateral hemispheres and forms the largest portion of the human brain. It presides over such processes as interpretation of sensation, rationality, decision making, memory, behavior, social and moral sense, and all aspects of behavior that places us in a category above the animal kingdom.

The cerebellum occupies the posterior cranial cavity of the skull. It is mainly involved in the control of skeletal muscular activity. An example would be the control of muscle tone and coordination during voluntary movement.

The brainstem forms the central portion of the brain and it consists of, from inferior to superior, the medulla (oblongata), pons,

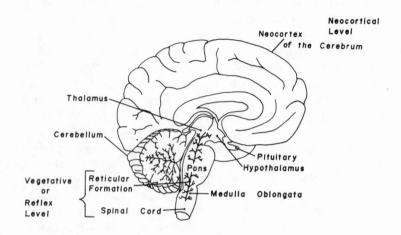

Figure 4

The human brain.

midbrain, and diencephalon. The medulla oblongata is a center that is mainly involved in the control of breathing, blood circulation, and heart rate. The pons consists of a network of neural pathways that sends information to several parts of the brain. The diencephalon includes the hypothalamus and the thalamus. The thalamus sends incoming information to various parts of the brain while the hypothalamus regulates such body functions as temperature, hunger, thirst, pleasure, and pain. The hypothalamus is also important in releasing several neurohumors or hormones which are responsible for the control of endocrine function in the body. This will be discussed in great detail later in the text. It is these two parts of the brain, the hypothalamus and the thalamus, that come into the foreground in a discussion of the stress response.

It must be remembered that the brain operates as a whole with its many interrelated parts; but from a functional point of view, the brain can be considered to be divided into three different but interrelated levels: the neocortical level, the limbic system, and the vegetative level (Figure 4).

The neocortex is that part of the brain which is the seat of higher mental functions and presides over such activities as rationality, imagination, and several of the other activities mentioned previously in the description of the cerebrum.

The limbic system is thought to consist of several neural structures such as the hypothalamus, thalamus, hippocampus, septum, and amygdala. This functional aspect of the brain is important because it seems to serve as the emotional or affective control center (MacLean, 1975). The pituitary gland is included since it serves as a master endocrine gland and receives messages from the hypothalamus. It is obvious that this level is important in a discussion of the stress response.

Finally the brainstem and reticular formation form the lowest functional level of the human brain. This level is concerned mainly with the maintenance of vegetative functions, such as vasomotor activity, respiration, heartbeat, etc. The reticular formation is a diffuse network which is centrally located throughout the brainstem. This network extends from the spinal cord on up to lower brain centers, such as the thalamus. It is a network which links both sensory and motor impulses, carrying information from various parts of the body to the brain, and vice versa. The functions of the reticular formation appear to be concerned with alerting or arousing the organism, and to coordinating reflex and voluntary movements. The reticular activating system is the name sometimes given to the reticular formation and its associated cortical fibers.

With regard to the spinal cord, it remains as a central pathway in which neurons send information to and from the brain and all other parts of the body.

In terms of the stress response, it is important to extend our discussion of brain function to the limbic system or emotional (affective) part of the brain. It is this part of the brain that plays an integral part in the stress response. Again, it is important to emphasize that no brain structure, or part of the brain, acts in isolation.

Emotional Brain

The emotional or affective brain, when considered in terms of function, is organized into an hierarchial system, starting from the mesencephalic midbrain nuclei, the reticular formation, to the hypothalamus, thalamus, limbic, and neocortical regions of the brain (Curtis et al., 1972).

Reticular Formation

The reticular formation receives information from the peripheral nervous system. It must be emphasized that only certain stimuli will trigger the reticular activating system which then performs its function in alerting the other portions of the brain. This is so because the organism has evolved a set of emotional responses which determine whether it will react to certain stimuli with anxiety or calm. The reticular activating system, along with the cortical subconscious, sorts out relevant information and alerts the organism. The outcome is that the central nervous system is able to function efficiently whenever a crisis situation arises.

Hypothalamus

Definite and well-organized emotional responses form the informational input that is received by the hypothalamus. The hypothalamus functions along with the thalamus to determine and establish the emotional state. These centers also work to coordinate and activate the appropriate cortical and subcortical centers.

Now, if a nonthreatening situation is presented, normal functioning continues within the organism. But if a stimulus is presented that is perceived as threatening, the elicitation of the stress response occurs, with its attendant autonomic nervous system end-organ effects. If the stimulus is perceived as a greater threat, the organism may respond with a more intense expression of emotion in eliciting the stress response. Here the end result may be one of increased physiological end-organ responses as a result of the recruitment of sympathetic end-organ activity. Once the stimulus is no longer perceived as a threat to the organism, there is a return, which may be somewhat delayed, to a balanced functioning between sympathetic and parasympathetic nervous systems.

Limbic Cortical Region

The limbic cortical region, upon receiving the hypothalamic emotional patterns, continues to expand upon and organize this information. The frontal cortex and, to a lesser degree, the temporal lobe with its information from the past, reviews the new information, sorts out the emotional and intellectual components, and exerts control by being excitatory or inhibitory.

PERIPHERAL NERVOUS SYSTEM

The peripheral nervous system is composed of all neurons that are not part of the central nervous system. It may be divided into two major nervous pathways, namely, the somatic and automatic nervous systems.

The somatic pathway is involved in impulse conduction which carries sensory and motor information to and from the central nervous system. The tissues that are innervated include the senses and the skeletal muscles.

The autonomic nervous system is that part of the peripheral nervous system which supplies motor fibers to smooth and cardiac muscles and glands. It is, in essence, concerned with the regulation of the internal environment of the body or, in other words, with the maintenance of homeostasis.

Autonomic Nervous System

The autonomic nervous system is composed of two distinct branches, namely, the sympathetic (thoracolumbar) and parasympathetic (craniosacral). Both of these divisions have anatomical as well as functional differences.

Anatomically, the differences in the two systems arise from their origin in the central nervous system. The sympathetic nerves originate in the spinal cord between the thoracic and lumbar spinal segments. On the other hand, the parasympathetic nerves have a few fibers which leave the CNS through several cranial nerves and a few sacral spinal nerves. It is safe to say that about 75 percent of all the parasympathetic fibers are in the vagus nerve which innervates several structures located in the thorax and abdominal regions of the body.

Unlike the peripheral processes of the somatic nervous system, which involve only a singe neuron between the brain, spinal cord, and effector organ, those of the autonomic nervous system involve two neurons (Figure 5). In the autonomic nervous system, the cell body of the first neuron is situated in the brain or spinal cord. This neuron then leaves the CNS, extending its axon to synapse with one or several other nerve fibers.

Figure 6 illustrates the sympathetic portion of the autonomic nervous system in terms of its gross and microscopic anatomy. As shown by the heavy lines, it can be seen that the segments T-1 through L-2 are the origin of the sympathetic fibers in the spinal cord. The preganglionic sympathetic fibers first pass into a paravertebral chain. These chains exist on either side of the spinal cord (only one is shown in the figure). From here the postganglionic sympathetic fibers pass into the various tissues and organs shown on the right side of the figure. Both preganglionic and postganglionic fibers are shown. On the other hand, the dashed lines represent postganglionic fibers in the gray rami of the spinal cord. These fibers send signals through spinal nerve transmission, to the organs and tissues illustrated on the left side of the figure, namely blood vessels, sweat glands, and pilo-erector muscles. (Guyton, 1981)

Figure 7 illustrates the same information for the parasympathetic nervous system. Its origin, in the cranial and sacral portions of the cord, is shown. However, for the parasympathetic system, the preganglionic fibers pass uninterrupted to the organ or tissue innervated. The preganglionic fibers synapse with the postganglionic neurons right within the walls of the organ being innervated. The short postganglionic fibers then innervate the various portions of the organ. (Guyton, 1981)

One can see that there is a marked contrast in the arrangement of the sympathetic and parasympathetic systems. The cell bodies of the postganglionic neurons of the sympathetic nervous system are

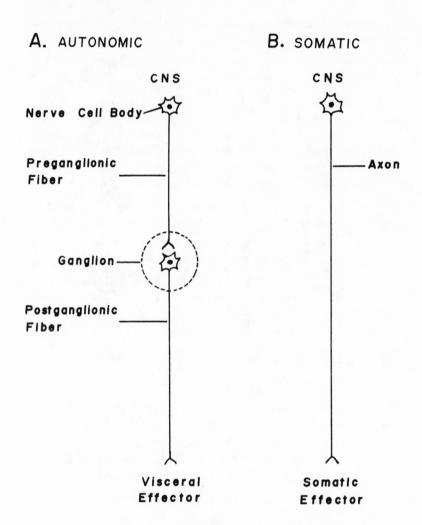

Figure 5

Schematic representation illustrating the difference between the somatic and autonomic neural pathways to effector organs.

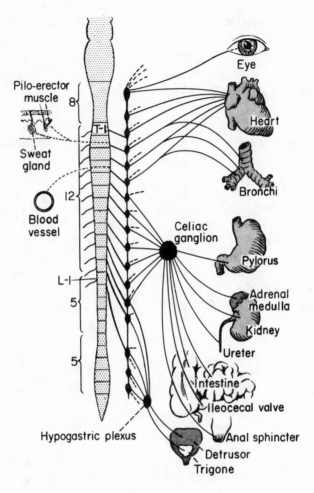

Figure 6

Sympathetic portion of the autonomic nervous system. Adapted from A.C. Guyton, *Textbook of Medical Physiology*, (6th ed.). Philadelphia: W.B. Saunders Co., 1981, p. 710.

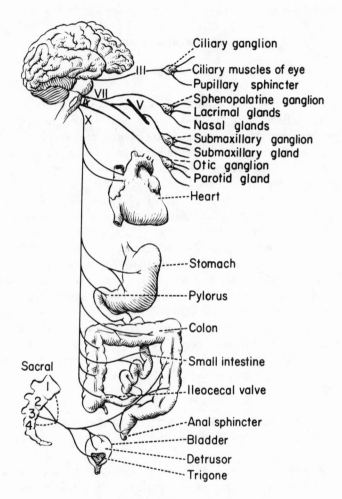

Figure 7

Parasympathetic portion of the autonomic nervous system. Adapted from A.C. Guyton, *Textbook of Medical Physiology*, (6th ed.). Philadelphia: W.B. Saunders Co., 1981, p. 711.

almost always located outside the organ being innervated either in chains or discrete ganglia, while those of the parasympathetic system are located in the innervated organ itself.

Autonomic Nervous System Activation

From a functional point of view, the autonomic nervous system controls basic body processes, as its name implies, which includes among other things, the regulation of heart rate, respiration, blood pressure, hormonal balance, metabolism, and reproduction.

We find that in times of stress the autonomic nervous system is activated, which serves to prepare the body to meet new demands placed upon it. This generally involves energy-expending processes. It is actually the sympathetic branch which functions in this respect. Its general effect on the organs in which it innervates, is one of arousal or escalation of activity. On the other hand, the parasympathetic branch of the autonomic nervous system is mainly concerned with restorative activities and the relaxation of the body. It acts to counterbalance the activity of the sympathetic nervous system in that it plays a role in slowing the body down or returning it to a resting level following an emergency response. The specific effects on the various systems of the body and on end-organ responses due to sympathetic and parasympathetic activation, are described and summarized in Table I.

PHYSIOLOGICAL EFFECTS OF SYMPATHETIC AND PARASYMPATHETIC ACTIVATION

A brief description of the physiological effects of autonomic activation on various systems of the body is given below.

Cardiovascular System

Heart

During the stress response, there is an increased sympathetic discharge, which results in an increase in myocardial contractility,

Organ	Effect of Sympathetic Stimulation	Effect of Parasympathetic Stimulation
Eye: Pupil	Dilated	Constricted
Ciliary muscle	Slight relaxation	Contracted
Glands: Nasal	Vasoconstriction and slight	Stimulation of thin, copious
Lacrimal	secretion	secretion (containing many enzymes
Parotid		for enzyme-secreting glands)
Submaxillary		
Gastric		
Pancreatic		
Sweat glands	Copious sweating (cholinergic)	None
Apocrine glands	Thick, odoriferous secretion	None
Heart: Muscle	Increased rate	Slowed rate
	Increased force of contraction	Decreased force of atrial contraction
Coronaries	Dilated (β_2); constricted (α)	Dilated
Lungs: Bronchi	Dilated	Constricted
Blood vessels	Mildly constricted	? Dilated
Gut: Lumen	Decreased peristalsis and tone	Increased peristalsis and tone
Sphincter	Increased tone	Relaxed
Liver	Glucose released	Slight glycogen synthesis
Gallbladder and bile ducts	Relaxed	Contracted
Kidney	Decreased output	None
Bladder: Detrusor	Relaxed	Excited
Trigone	Excited	Relaxed
Penis	Ejaculation	Erection
Systemic blood vessels:		
Abdominal	Constricted	None
Muscle	Constricted (adrenergic α)	None
	Dilated (adrenergic β)	
	Dilated (cholinergic)	
Skin	Constricted	None
Blood: Coagulation	Increased	None
Glucose	Increased	None
Basal metabolism	Increased up to 100%	None
Adrenal cortical secretion	Increased	None
Mental activity	Increased	None
Piloerector muscles	Excited	None
Skeletal muscle	Increased glycogenolysis	None
	Increased strength	

Table I

Autonomic Effects of Various Organs of the Body. Adapted from A.C. Guyton, *Textbook of Medical Physiology*, (6th ed.). Philadelphia: W.B. Saunders Co., 1981, p. 715.

heart rate, and metabolism of the heart. On the other hand, parasympathetic discharge will decrease the above.

Arterial Pressure

Sympathetic stimulation increases the cardiac output and causes a general vascular constriction. This vascular constriction will increase total peripheral resistance and thereby cause an elevation in the blood pressure. On the other hand, parasympathetic stimulation decreases the pumping action of the heart, thereby contributing to a lower blood pressure.

Upon elicitation of the stress response, it is sympathetic stimulation that becomes prominent.

Systemic Vasculature

Sympathetic stimulation causes most of the vasculature of the body to constrict, especially the vasculature of the periphery (skin) and of the abdominal region. During the stress response, this peripheral vasoconstriction is seen as a blanching of the skin or a shunting of the blood away from the periphery. Parasympathetic activity generally does not exert any influence on the systemic vasculature, although a few isolated cases have been observed where parasympathetic influence was more prominent than sympathetic influence.

Gastrointestinal System

Under normal conditions, the gastrointestinal system is not much affected by the stimulation of the sympathetic nervous system. But in some conditions, an increase in sphincter tone and an inhibition of peristaltic movement can occur with sympathetic overactivation. The outcome is a slow movement of food substance through the gastrointestinal tract. Blood flow to the gastrointestinal tract is also influenced by the sympathetic nervous system. An increase in sympathetic activity causes the blood to be shunted away from the gastrointestinal tract and therefore results in a decrease in the blood flow to the digestive organs.

Parasympathetic activity can cause the gastrointestinal tract to relax the sphincters and will increase G.I. peristaltic movement, which in turn, will increase the transfer of food substance down the gastrointestinal tract.

Both of these responses have been observed during elicitation of the stress response.

Respiratory System

The sympathetic and parasympathetic systems both exert rather mild effects on the lungs. The sympathetic system will dilate the bronchi and constrict the blood vessels, while the parasympathetic system can cause the opposite effect (constrict the bronchi and dilate the blood vessels).

Various Glands of the Body

Sweat glands

Sympathetic discharge results in an increased amount of activity from the sweat glands, while parasympathetic stimulation exerts no influence on these glands. Upon elicitation of the stress response, increased perspiration occurs, along with an increased skin conductivity or decreased skin resistance. One can use measured values of conductance or resistance to assess arousal states.

Apocrine glands

Apocrine glands are secretory glands which lose part of their cytoplasm during their secretory activity. Certain sweat glands can be included in this category. These glands respond to sympathetic stimulation in much the same way as the sweat glands described above.

The nasal, salivary, lacrimal, and many gastrointestinal glands are apocrine glands and as such can be stimulated to secrete large amounts of fluid in response to increased parasympathetic activity. As far as the gastrointestinal tract is concerned, the parasympathetic nervous system exerts its main influence on the mouth and stomach portions of the tract. Sympathetic stimulation on the other hand constricts the vasculature which supplies the above mentioned glands. This then decreases their overall secretory capability.

Eye

Sympathetic activity results in a pupillary dilation while parasympathetic activity constricts the pupil. During periods of arousal or excitement, the sympathetics are stimulated, which results in an increase in the pupillary opening. This phenomenon is generally seen during the stress response.

Brain

The process of mentation and alertness will increase dramatically during sympathetic discharge.

Muscle

During sympathetic discharge (as seen during the "fight or flight" response), muscle strength is increased.

Other Structures of the Body

In general, sympathetic stimulation exerts an inhibitory influence on the ducts of the gallbladder, liver, ureter, and bladder, while parasympathetic system stimulation excites these structures.

Metabolism

During the stress response, the sympathetic nervous system plays a dominant role in metabolism. Sympathetic stimulation increases basal metabolic rate, causes an increase in blood levels of glucose, causes hepatic glucose release and an increase in glycogenolysis (glycogen breakdown) in muscle. These effects typically occur during the elicitation of the stress response.

PARASYMPATHETIC EFFECTS OF THE STRESS RESPONSE

It has been stated previously that the physiological mechanisms which underlie the stress response initiate with the arousal of the sympathetic portion of the autonomic nervous system. This is generally the case in many instances. However, there are circumstances in which parasympathetic activity comes into prominence as a result of the elicitation of the stress response. This results in physiological dysfunctioning characterized by specific unpleasant side effects. Stress-induced sympathetic arousal accompanied by parasympathetic activation has been demonstrated by the work of

Gellhorn (1968), Engle (1971), and Carruthers and Taggart (1973).

Let us consider a case in point. There is a central nervous system condition called syncope, more commonly referred to as fainting. This is described as a transient form of unconsciousness during which the person falls to the ground as a result of cerebral anoxia. This condition may be due to a deficiency in the supply of blood reaching the brain because of 1) disturbances in cardiac function or cardiac failure, 2) peripheral circulatory failure, or 3) alteration in the quality of blood as in hyperventilation or hypoglycemia.

Some of the predisposing factors which result in the onset of this condition include: fatigue, pain, poor ventilation, prolonged standing, nausea, and a variety of emotional disturbances. All of these factors can be labelled as stressful conditions, or as stressors.

Psychogenically induced fainting has been shown to be difficult to study scientifically in the laboratory but it certainly is not an uncommon occurrence. For example, fainting subsequent to or in anticipation of witnessing a surgical operation for the first time, or engaging in combat, can be attributed to psychogenic causes.

The initial physiological response as a reaction to these stressful stimuli may at first be one of sympathetic arousal, as generally happens, and secondarily, increased parasympathetic activity. As an aspect of increased sympathetic activation, it is known that the blood is channeled away from the periphery and a large amount is pooled in the muscular system due to the increased vasodilatation that occurs there. The organism is then prepared to respond to a threat (the "fight or flight" response). This combination coupled with a decrease in mobility will lead to a decrease in venous return. This, in turn, coupled with an increase in parasympathetic stimulation, such as an increase in vagus nerve activity, a decrease in blood pressure and a decrease in blood flow to the heart and brain, may all contribute to the end-organ response seen in syncope. As described, this condition may be the result of the elicitation of the stress response which is first characterized by an initial sympathetic arousal, followed by an increase in parasympathetic activity. Here, the prominent parasympathetic effect is increased vagal activity, decreased blood pressure and heart rate.

Another example of stress-induced parasympathetic activity is seen in some subjects who respond with an increased muscle tone and increased peristalsis in the gastrointestinal tract, instead of a sympathetic decreased tone and decreased peristalsis. Such subjects in this state experience an irregular and rapid movement of fluid down the gastrointestinal tract. Because of the decreased contact time of the fluid along the walls of the tract, a minimum amount of fluid is reabsorbed. The outcome is an increase in the frequency of bowel evacuation having a more or less fluid consistency.

On the other hand, sympathetic arousal precipitates a decrease in tone and in peristaltic movement, the outcome of which is sluggish activity of the bowels. Predisposing factors may include diet, inflammation or irritation of the intestines, infections, and psychogenic factors such as worry, fear, and anxiety.

Another instance of heightened parasympathetic activity may be described. It is known that emotional reactivity to certain stimuli may result in the familiar peripheral reddening of the skin, or blushing of the face. This is due to localized vasodilation. It is known that parasympathetic activity in general does not exert any influence on the systemic vasculature. There are a few isolated cases in which systemic parasympathetic influence may be observed. In this case, certain localized facial regions respond to such parasympathetic activity.

Another phenomenon mediated by the parasympathetic nervous system is weeping. It may be stated that emotional reactivity either to a large or small extent has been known to induce psychological weeping.

Still another disturbance mediated by the parasympathetic nervous system is that of bronchoconstriction. Bronchospasm is a condition described by a reversible narrowing of the bronchi and bronchioles of the lungs. It is familiarly described as an asthmatic attack and can be psychogenically induced or can occur as a result of local irritation of the mucosal lining of the respiratory tract by foreign substances, such as pollen or other environmental pollutants. Since it is known that bronchiolar vasoconstrictor reflexes are present, the possibility exists that the parasympathetic nervous system via the vagus nerve may, at least in part, play a role in mediating such an attack.

It was mentioned previously that the primary emphasis of the parasympathetic portion of the autonomic nervous system is one of relaxation of the body, returning it to resting levels following an emergency response. However, some subjects in responding to chronic stress, in the long term, may exaggerate this response and manifest such conditions as generalized lethargy and overweight coupled with various states of depression. These states are characteristically parasympathetic in nature and may be a result of increased frequency or heightened parasympathetic activity over long periods of time. The physiological mechanisms underlying these conditions are not at present known. However, it may be speculated that in this case, a hormonal mechanism may also be involved in the long term expression of the stress response. Stress-induced depression of thyroid stimulating hormone activity from the anterior pituitary may influence the thyroid hormonal output of the thyroid gland in the long term, resulting in an hypometabolic, depressed state for the organism. The symptoms described above are analogous to the symptomology developed in a hypothyroid individual.

The description above cites only a few examples of heightened parasympathetic activity elicited as a result of stress reactivity. This by no means exhausts the number of examples that could be included. Needless to say, much work remains to be done in this area, particularly in terms of investigating the physiological mechanisms involved. Also, due to the vast number of individual differences entailed, as well as the vast number of ways of reacting to stressful stimuli, it is not possible to predict when, where, and with whom, long-term increased parasympathetic activity will be more pronounced, as compared to increased sympathetic activity. For a more comprehensive discussion of the simultaneous activation of the parasympathetic and sympathetic branches of the autonomic nervous system, refer to the work of Darrow, 1943.

NEUROTRANSMITTERS OF THE
AUTONOMIC NERVOUS SYSTEM

As was previously mentioned during a general discussion of neuronal pathways, impulse transmission from neuron to neuron is chemical; that is, it occurs via the release of a neurotransmitter substance. Transmission from preganglionic to postganglionic neurons in the autonomic nervous system occurs by means of the release of the neurotransmitter substance, acetylcholine. In fact, all preganglionic neurons of both the sympathetic and parasympathetic nervous systems release this same neurotransmitter and are therefore said to be cholinergic. Also, acetylcholine or acetylcholine-like substances will excite both the sympathetic and parasympathetic postganglionic neurons.

The postganglionic nerve fibers which encompass the parasympathetic nervous system are also cholinergic. On the other hand, we find that the postganglionic fibers of the sympathetic nervous system release norepinephrine as a neurotransmitter. These nerve terminals are referred to as adrenergic. The exception to the rule are the postganglionic sympathetic fibers to the sweat glands and to a few blood vessels, which are cholinergic. So, in general, postganglionic or terminal sympathetic nerve endings are adrenergic and release or secrete norepinephrine, while the postganglionic or terminal parasympathetic nerve endings are cholinergic and secrete acetylcholine. As a result of activation, the release of these hormones then mediate the various sympathetic and parasympathetic effects seen as end-organ responses. The molecular structure of these hormones are shown in Figure 8.

The time sequence of adrenergic or cholinergic release from nerve endings and activation is of short duration. For example, after release from adrenergic nerve endings, norepinephrine remains active in a tissue or organ for only a few seconds. This can be compared to the release of this same substance along with epinephrine from the adrenal medulla. The secretions of the adrenal medulla reach the end-organs by means of the bloodstream. With adrenal medullary secretion, both of these hormones remain active in the body for approximately one-half of a minute, followed by an attenuation of activity for one to several minutes. This demonstrates the rapid phenomenon of neurotransmitter re-uptake in the nervous system compared to endocrine hormonal degradation in the other tissues of the body.

This phenomenon has implication for the stress response. Upon elicitation of the stress response, it is the activity of the autonomic

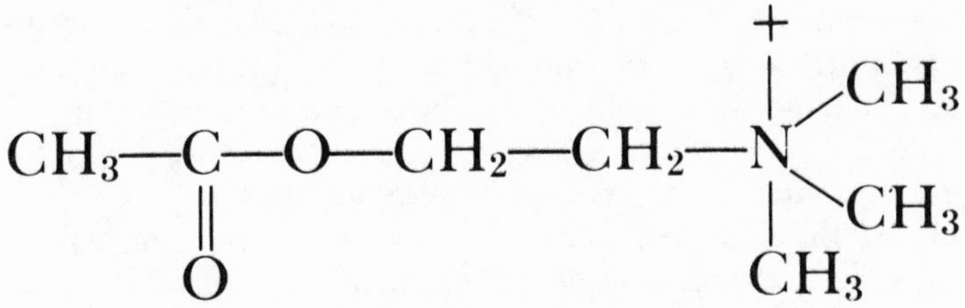

$$CH_3-\underset{\underset{O}{\|}}{C}-O-CH_2-CH_2-\overset{+}{N}\underset{CH_3}{\overset{CH_3}{<}}$$

CH₃

Acetylcholine

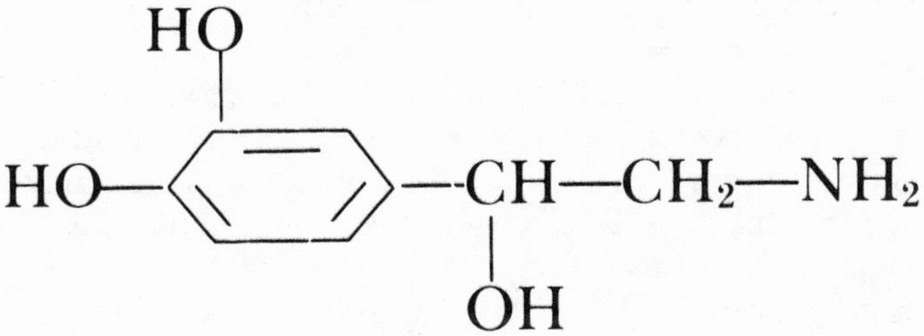

$$HO-\langle\!\!\!\rangle-\underset{\underset{OH}{|}}{CH}-CH_2-NH_2$$

with HO on top of ring

Norepinephrine

Figure 8

Chemical structures of the autonomic nervous system neurotransmitters, acetylcholine and norepinephrine.

nervous system which is at first pronounced. This is followed by activation of the various other endocrine axes.

EFFECTOR ORGAN RECEPTORS

The manner in which the neurotransmitter substance activates its target tissue, is first to react with a specific receptor substance (or receptor site) on the effector organ. This is analogous to the way hormones influence their target tissues. They react specifically with a receptor site which, for example, may be located in the cell membranes of their target cells. For the neurotransmitter substance, the receptor is almost always located in the cell membrane. The mechanism of receptor interaction may be described as follows: when the neurotransmitter first reacts with the receptor, it alters the chemical nature of the receptor, which can lead to subsequent cellular changes, such as alteration of cellular membrane permeability, or activation of membrane enzymes. This in turn can lead to changes in intracellular enzyme activity and cellular chemical reactions. The final result is the specific physiological response produced by the effector organ. This is discussed in further detail in the next chapter.

Through drug studies, it has been found that acetylcholine activates two types of receptors, namely, the muscarinic and nicotinic receptors. The cells containing muscarinic receptors are found in those organs innervated by cholinergic neurons of both the sympathetic and parasympathetic nervous systems. On the other hand, nicotinic receptors are located at the neuromuscular junction of skeletal muscle and between preganglionic and postganglionic fibers of both the sympathetic and parasympathetic nervous systems.

Scientific investigators have identified two different types of adrenergic receptors, alpha (α) and beta (β) receptors. The two catecholamines secreted by the adrenal medulla excite these receptors with differing sensitivity. For example, epinephrine excites, with almost equal intensity, the effector organs which contain alpha receptors and those which contain beta receptors. On the other hand, the effector organs containing alpha receptors are excited by norepinephrine to a much greater extent than those effector organs which contain beta receptors. Thus the excitation of various organs by the catecholamines is a function of the types of receptors which they contain. Further, the activity of the effector organ can be either excitatory or inhibitory. The implication for the stress response is obvious. One can see that as a result of this phenomenon, end-organ responsivity during stress can be quite varied. Table II illustrates the types of adrenergic receptors, along with their physiolog-

Alpha Receptor	Beta Receptor
Vasoconstriction	Vasodilatation (β_2)
Iris dilatation	Cardioacceleration (β_1)
Intestinal relaxation	Increased myocardial strength (β_1)
Intestinal sphincter contraction	Intestinal relaxation (β_2)
	Uterus relaxation (β_2)
Pilomotor contraction	Bronchodilatation (β_2)
Bladder sphincter contraction	Calorigenesis (β_2)
	Glycogenolysis (β_2)
	Lipolysis (β_1)
	Bladder relaxation (β_2)

Table II

Relationship of Adrenergic Receptors and Function. Adapted from A.C. Guyton, *Textbook of Medical Physiology*, (6th ed.). Philadelphia: W.B. Saunders Co., 1981, p. 714.

ical responses. More recent research has demonstrated that both the alpha and beta receptors are further subdivided (alpha$_1$, alpha$_2$, beta$_1$, and beta$_2$). Various drug studies have uncovered the diversity in the alpha and beta receptors, as evidenced by the fact that certain drugs activate certain receptors and not others. Other receptors have also recently been discoverd such as the gamma receptor and further investigations may yet reveal the existance of several other types of receptors.

SUMMARY

In this section we have outlined the basic cellular mechanisms involved in the process of neural transmission. The human nervous system, comprised of the central and peripheral nervous systems, and the positions they hold during the elicitation of the stress response, was described. As part of the peripheral and central nervous systems, and in view of its role in the stress response, the basic anatomy and physiology of the autonomic nervous system was reviewed. Finally, a brief outline of the concept of neurotransmitter substance, along with the neurotransmitters of the autonomic nervous system, was presented.

In terms of the central nervous system, a study of the final common pathways through which the brain controls the endocrine and autonomic nervous systems is certainly of significance, and deserves continued investigation. It is both these systems that play a dominate role in the stress response. Within the recent past much has certainly been learned about these systems, including their participation in mediating human reactivity to changing environments. These studies have led to the characterization of several hypothalamic hormones, also known as hypothalamic releasing factors, which will be discussed in the next chapter. Also, recent investigations of brain receptors have led to studies of neuropeptides, which is indeed of importance and significance in understanding brain function and behavior, and may play a role in the elicitation of the stress response.

CHAPTER 3

The
Stress Response

The stress response is evoked initially by a stimulus which may be either external or internal to the organism, and which is perceived by the organism to be a threat. If the stimulus is internal, it may be evoked by a cognitive and/or affective state, or an internal physical sensation. If the stimulus is external, it must be received by sensory receptors of the peripheral nervous system. Upon sensory receptor stimulation, the information is sent up sensory neural pathways toward the brain. These signals reach the reticular formation and are then relayed on to the limbic system and may be integrated with other emotional states which are stored there. The information is also sent on up other neural pathways that reach the cortical levels of the brain where an analytical interpretation of the stimulus occurs. The information present is now both rationally and perhaps emotionally integrated. This information is sent back via signal conduction to the limbic system. Here an emotional arousal will probably result if the cortical-limbic or rational-emotional interpretation of the stimulus induces a perception of a threat or a danger.

If the stress response is not evoked initially by an external stimulus, then the same cortical and limbic integration of information occurs, but the sensory receptor activation step is bypassed.

The important point again to emphasize here is that the stress response which is evoked is not a result of the stimulus under consideration, but is actually a direct result of the cognitive interpretation and/or emotional arousal of the organism. In terms of the reactions which occur in the body, the stress response itself is comprised of over 1,400 physiochemical changes (Wilson & Schneider, 1981). All of these changes can be activated to varying degrees and at various periods of time. As described in the next sections, these reactions are initiated by the nervous system and then carried through by neuroendocrine mechanisms.

PATHWAYS ACTIVATED BY THE STRESS RESPONSE

There are two main physiological axes or pathways that are activated upon elicitation of the stress response. These two axes are the neural and neuroendocrine systems.

Autonomic Nervous System Activation

The first major axis or pathway which is activated during the elicitation of the stress response is that of the autonomic nervous system.

The autonomic nervous system can be activated by stimuli from the central nervous system or by external stimuli impinging upon sensory receptors, which result in transference of information to the central nervous system.

To be more specific, activation of the autonomic nervous system by the central nervous system occurs, in general, by centers located in the spinal cord, brainstem and hypothalamus. Also, lower brain centers may receive information from portions of the cerebral cortex and limbic system, thereby exerting an influence on the autonomic nervous system.

On the other hand, external stimuli may excite sensory receptors which send signals from sensory organs that travel by means of nerve conduction to enter the spinal cord, brainstem, and hypothalamus. These structures in turn can transmit responses back to autonomically innervated effector organs and thereby influence autonomic activity.

More specifically, in terms of the stress response and autonomic activation, the signals which have been encoded as threatening or endangering reach the hypothalamus from cortical and limbic structures. The sympathetic portion of the autonomic nervous system is then activated by those signals with the encoded information that emerge from the posterior portion of the hypothalamus. The parasympathetic portion is activated by those signals emerging from the anterior portion of the hypothalamus. As described previously, the sympathetic neural pathways which originate in the posterior hypothalamus descend down the cord through the thoracic and lumbar regions of the cord, ultimately innervating specific end-organs by the spinal nerves. In like manner, the parasympathetic pathways, which originate in the anterior hypothalamus, travel down the cord and the spinal nerves emerge through the cranial and sacral regions of the spinal cord innervating specific end-organs. In this regard, it is clear that the hypothalamus is one of the major areas of the brain responsible for regulating autonomic nervous system activity.

Sympathetic Activation

The immediate effect of sympathetic activation is overall body arousal. The purpose is to allow the body to act over and above its normal everyday functioning. For example, it provides the body with an elevated heart rate, increased circulation, increased oxygen supply, increased metabolism, and energy to handle a threatening or endangering situation. The end-organ effects of sympathetic activation are reviewed in Table 1. In general, sympathetic stimulation enhances overall body arousal, stimulating the organs that are needed in the "fight or flight" response, and inhibiting those that are not required. Prolonged stimulation of these organs can result in an altered physiological state which could, in the long term, lead to a stress-related disorder.

Parasympathetic Activation

Stimulation of the parasympathetic system has the opposite effect. For example, heart rate slows, pupils constrict, and blood vessels dilate (refer to Table 1). In general, the effects of parasympathetic activation are concerned with slowing down the organism and are more restorative in nature. Perhaps it can be stated that parasympathetic activity is heightened in an organism that is satisfied and contented.

It must be remembered that most organs of the body are innervated by the sympathetic and parasympathetic systems. Many times these two systems act wholly as a unit. Also, whenever any part of one system is activated, it turns out that all or most of that system is activated.

However, there are many instances in which both the sympathetic and parasympathetic systems do not act in this manner. For example, upon elicitation of the stress response, an individual may react with only heightened activity in an isolated end-organ innervated by the sympathetic nervous system, such as the sweat glands, resulting in increased sweating. The stress response may also activate several end-organ systems. Heightened parasympathetic activation can also result in isolated end-organ activity as well as multiple activity in specific groups of organs. Figure 9 summarizes the initial physiological axis that is activated during the stress response.

Pathway A is heightened during the stress response, which is mainly sympathetic activation resulting in overall heightened arousal of the organism. As discussed previously, there may be some parasympathetic end-organ stress reactions.

The effect on end-organ activity of the autonomic nervous system activation during the stress response is quite rapid. This is so because of the nature of neural transmission, since all of the pathways involved are neural. The effects are not long-lasting due to the rapid degradation and re-uptake of the neurotransmitter substance. Also, there is a finite amount of neurotransmitter which is available for release. The stores of neurotransmitter can eventually become exhausted under intense and constant stimulation. Therefore, in order to maintain the arousal state for longer periods of time, additional physiological components are activated.

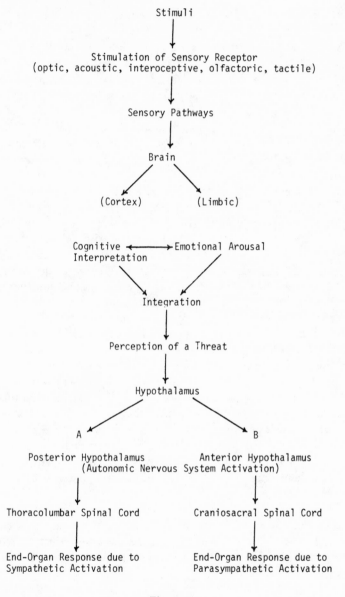

Figure 9
The initial phase of activation of the stress response.

Fight or Flight Response.

Cannon was the first to describe the "fight or flight" response (Cannon 1911, 1914). The "fight or flight" response prepares the body to react to a threat or danger. The body is prepared for heightened muscular activity so that it may either fight or flee the perceived threat or danger.

The "fight or flight" response describes the next pathway or axis that is activated by the stress response. This response is the result of both neural and endocrine activity and hence is neuroendocrine in nature.

The main endocrine organ involved is the adrenal medulla.

The origin of the "fight or flight" response lies in the dorsomedialamygdalar complex (Roldan et al. 1974). From here, the neural pathways pass to the lateral and posterior portions of the hypothalamus, continuing downward to the thoracic regions, and on to the adrenal medulla. Sympathetic stimulation of the adrenal medulla results in the release of the catecholamines; epinephrine (adrenaline) and norepinephrine (noradrenaline).

Figure 10 summarizes this phase or physiological axis that is activated during the stress response. The initial activation of the brain structures, along with cortical and affective integration, occurs but is omitted here, for the sake of simplicity (Figure 9).

The catecholamines intensify or increase the general adrenergic activity of the sympathetic nervous system. In essence, they mimic sympathetic activity. However, since they are hormones that are secreted, a small period of time is required for their release. The outcome is an approximate half-minute delay in their onset of action. They also prolong the effects of the adrenergic sympathetic response; hence they represent a more chronic phase of the stress response.

An increase in secretion of these medullary hormones can exert pronounced effects on the physiology of the organism. The cardiovascular system, respiratory system, gastrointestinal system, central nervous system, the blood, and metabolism are markedly affected by these hormones.

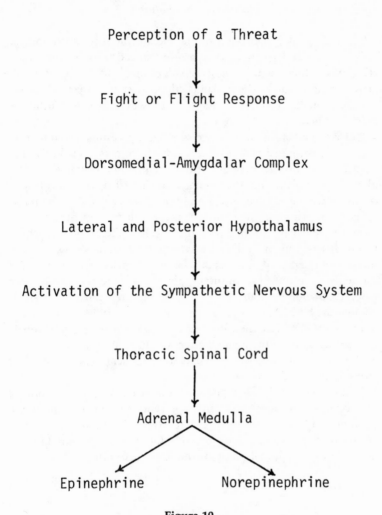

Figure 10

The intermediate phase of activation of the stress response.

Endocrine Activation

The final phase, incorporating the most prolonged physiological activity of the stress response, is a result of activation of the endocrine axis, which includes various endocrine glands of the body. A general description of these glands, along with the effects of stress, is offered in the following chapters. However, a brief outline is presented here.

Chronic elicitation of the stress response results in endocrine activation. A longer time is required, both for endocrine hormonal release and transport throughout the circulation. Several endocrine glands are involved, but the main glands that are directly influenced by stress are the adrenal cortex and the pituitary glands. The highest point of origin, in the brain, for these endocrine glands, appears to be the septal-hippocampal complex (Henry & Stephens, 1977). From this region, neural pathways transmit signals down to the median eminence of the hypothalamus. The hypothalamus then influences the anterior pituitary gland to secrete its respective trophic hormones, many of which are elevated during the stress response. These hormones, in turn, influence various target organs in the body to secrete their hormones. The target organ hormones, thus released, have the general effect of changing the environment within the organism, so that adaptation to heightened arousal or stress is accomodated.

In summary, this final phase of the stress response is one of endocrine organ activation and represents the most chronic and prolonged physiological response to stress. It requires a stronger stimulus of activation, as compared to the stimulus required for the activation of the initial phase of the stress response.

GENERAL ADAPTATION SYNDROME

Hans Selye (1951) advanced the theory that the body responds to stressors, the name given to a wide variety of nonspecific stimuli, by a more or less consistent series of physiological responses which he termed the general adaptation syndrome (GAS). The GAS, is in reality, a theoretical concept used to describe the series of nervous and endocrine gland activities that take place during the chronic phase of stress reactivity. The GAS is more than a response to stress. It is a process which occurs, permitting the body to counteract stressful stimuli in the most effective way possible. The GAS is divided into three phases:

(1) Alarm reaction: a stressor causes an initial activation of the body's defense mechanism. What ensues is a complex physiological response involving several interacting systems within the body. The alarm reaction is basically characterized by the release of adrenal medullary and cortical hormones into the bloodstream. In summary, most investigators today consider the alarm phase of the GAS to be the sympathetic response known as the "fight or flight" response with subsequent release of epiniphrine into the bloodstream due to adrenal medullary activation. This is followed by an ACTH-adrenal cortical response.

(2) Stage of resistance: There is a dramatic reduction in alarm reactions, as full resistance to the stressor is developed. Here it is an attempt on the part of the body to maintain homeostasis in the presence of the stressor which initiated the alarm reaction. Cortisol secretion is elevated, and the body is functioning at heightened levels. If the stressor prevails, then the mechanisms involved in supporting this stage of resistance will weaken.

(3) Stage of exhaustion: Here, the endocrine activity is heightened. High circulating levels of cortisol begin to produce pronounced effects on the circulatory, digestive, immune, and other systems of the body. Shock, ulcers, and lowered resistance to infection may begin to appear as the adaptation can no longer prevail. Indeed, in many cases, this experience can prove lethal to the organism.

SUMMARY

This section has described the stress response in terms of the two basic physiological pathways or axes that are activated. The sequential timing of activation of these axes was also delineated.

The most rapid response occurs with the activation of the autonomic nervous system (sympathetic arousal). This is purely a neural pathway, culminating in neural innervation of end-organs. The neuroendocrine activation (sympathetic stimulation of the adrenal medulla) contributes to the intermediate effects of stress. This activation is also known as the "fight or flight" response. Finally, activation of the neuroendocrine axes, comprising several endocrine glands, accounts for the most prolonged and chronic phase of the stress response. The temporal delay is built into the neuroendocrine component of the stress response, since the dependence is on hormonal release and transport throughout the circulatory system. Overlap may occur between the various neural and neuroendocrine mechanisms. Finally, the GAS was presented and was described as a way in which the endocrine activation phase could be extended into the process of adaptation by the organism to chronic stress.

The physiological axes of the stress response show a large amount of built-in variation. Not all end-organ responses occur with each activation. Also, there is a large amount of individual variation in end-organ response at the organism level superimposed upon the diversity of responses at the end-organ level. One can see that the end result of physiological activation during the stress response is structured along a hierarchy of complexity. However, to ease the complexity of the situation somewhat, evidence does exist to demonstrate that some individuals are predisposed to exhibit specific end-organ reactivity in response to certain stressors. Also, it is well known that, in general, individuals differ in the degree in which they respond to physiological activation by various stimuli. The variation in the degree of physiological activation as well as the length of time these same individuals require to return to baseline, that is, to pre-stimulus levels, also differs. As noted previously, different stimuli arouse different individuals with varying degrees of intensity.

In addition to this, there are the problems that one encounters when measuring these differences in physiological activation between individuals. These problems of measurement are much greater between individuals than those which one would encounter when measuring differences within an individual. Individual differences exist in the case where, in the presence of the same stimulus, one individual may respond with maximum reactivity in one end-organ or system, for example, the cardiovascular system, while another individual may respond with maximum reactivity in another end-organ or system such as the digestive system. In order to assess and draw any conclusions with regard to individual differences in reactivity, a statistical analysis based on a sampling of responses from many systems would therefore be required. Observations made, not only in humans, but in many other species, demonstrate individual differences in patterns of reactivity within the various species studied. For a more comprehensive review of this topic, the reader is referred to Lacey & Lacey, 1958 (a), Lacey & Lacey, 1958 (b) and Duffy, 1962.

CHAPTER 4

Endocrinology

GENERAL DISCUSSION

In presenting this section, the attempt has been made to avoid needless complexity and to present a clear but general description of the endocrine system. In order to understand the physiological changes which occur upon elicitation of the stress response, it is necessary to obtain a basic knowledge of the endocrine system in terms of its function.

As discussed previously, upon elicitation of the stress mechanism of the body, the endocrine system is highly activated and its altered hormonal secretions further influence other physiological functions. The endocrine system is important because it represents the most chronic and prolonged physiological response to stress. The endocrine system of the body functions along with the nervous system in governing bodily processes in order to maintain homeostatic control. In particular, the endocrine system, with its array of many hormones, is primarily concerned with general processes such as growth, metabolism, and sexual differentiation.

While the nervous system and endocrine system work together, they function entirely differently. The nervous system operates by means of nerve impulse transmission between nerves, muscles, and glands. The activity of the nervous system causes muscles to contract and glands to secrete. The tissue and end-organ response time is quite rapid after transmission. On the other hand, the glands of the endocrine system secrete hormones, often referred to as chemical messengers, into the blood. They are then transmitted to specific target tissues and organs by means of the circulation. It must be noted that the blood has easy access to body cells and reaches all the tissues and organs of the body. The main effect here of the activity of the endocrine system is to cause metabolic changes in specific organs and tissues. In contrast to the nervous system, endocrine hormonal activation generally takes much longer, requiring minutes, hours, or days for end-organ response. Hormonal activity may then persist for a considerable period of time, whereas the effects produced by the nervous system are generally quite brief.

HORMONES AND THEIR ACTIONS

The endocrine glands of the body secrete hormones which are released directly into the circulation surrounding the gland cells. This is in contrast to the other glands of the body, often referred to as exocrine glands. The secretions of the exocrine glands pass directly into a duct rather than directly into the bloodstream. The secreted hormones of the endocrine glands are then transported to various target tissues and organs of the body. Generally, a particular hormone often exerts its influence on a specific tissue. This tissue is termed its target tissue. The resultant physiological effect produced by the hormone is quite specific. Also, a particular hormone may affect more than just one tissue and influence several or all cells of the body. Figure 11 depicts the major endocrine glands of the body.

CHEMISTRY, MEASUREMENT, AND CONCENTRATIONS OF HORMONES

There are two basic types of hormones: 1) proteins or protein derivatives such as amino acids, and 2) steroids.

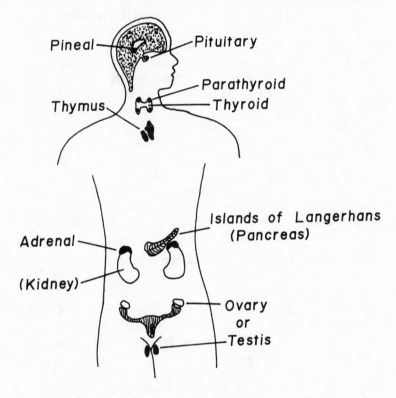

Figure 11
Major endocrine glands of the body.

For example, the hormones of the anterior pituitary, pancreas, and parathyroid glands are proteins. On the other hand, steroid hormones include those hormones secreted by the adrenal cortex, the ovary, and the testis.

Most endocrine glands continuously secrete hormones in amounts determined by bodily requirements. However, most hormones are generally present in the blood and/or tissues in extremely minute amounts. The concentration of a specific hormone can be as low as one nanogram per milliliter (10^{-9}/ml). Because of these low concentrations, it is not possible to measure hormones in the bloodstream by usual chemical means. Therefore, the two specific methods which are used today to measure hormonal concentrations, are bioassay and radioactive competitive binding. A discussion of these methods can be found in most physiology or biochemistry textbooks.

SECRETION OF HORMONES

Hormone secretion occurs because of stimuli that are generally either nervous or chemical in origin. An example of nervous control would be one of direct innervation. This occurs through fibers of the autonomic nervous system, which results in rapid hormonal secretion caused by nerve impulses. Sympathetic innervation of the adrenal medulla, and hypothalamic control of hormonal release from the posterior pituitary are good examples. On the other hand, an example of hormonal release because of chemical stimuli occurs during hypothalamic secretion of releasing factors (hormones) which in turn influence the anterior pituitary to secrete its hormones into the circulation.

OTHER FACTORS THAT INFLUENCE HORMONAL SECRETIONS

Blood levels of certain metabolites or organic substances influence certain hormonal secretions. For example, blood levels of glucose influence pancreatic hormonal secretion. Blood levels of certain inorganic substances also influence hormonal secretions. A good example of this would be the levels of blood calcium influencing the secretions of parathyroid and calcitonin hormones.

The osmolality or osmotic pressure of the blood can also influence hormonal secretions. The hormone directly involved here would be antidiuretic hormone (ADH) also known as vasopressin.

MECHANISM OF HORMONAL FEEDBACK CONTROL

Secretion of hormones is regulated by feedback control mechanisms. Consider this example: If hormone X is responsible for the secretion of hormone Y (i.e., as X increases, Y increases), then as the concentration of Y continues to increase in the bloodstream or in the tissues, the concentration of X begins to decrease. This is an example of a negative feedback control mechanism. The hormones of the anterior pituitary and their target tissue hormones exhibit this type of relationship. There are also examples in the endocrine system of positive feedback. The feedback control principle can be an example of homeostatic cybernetic control.

To summarize, hormonal secretion is governed by many various and diverse factors, all of which produce normal physiological functioning. As shall be seen subsequently in the text, the elicitation of the stress response has a pronounced effect on the endocrine system, producing changes in hormonal secretion, which result in an altered physiological state.

MECHANISM OF ACTION OF HORMONES

Hormones function to control the activity of certain target tissues. They may control this activity in a variety of ways. For example, hormones may change the chemical reactions occurring within cells, or even alter the permeability properties of their target cell membranes to certain substances. The different hormones achieve these effects by two general mechanisms:

(1) Hormone molecules can combine with specific receptor sites located at the level of the cell membranes of target cells. Once this hormone-receptor combination has been made, an enzyme, adenyl cyclase, located within the membrane is activated. Adenylate cyclase is stimulated directly then by specific hormones arriving from the bloodstream. This activation causes the formation of cyclic $3'$, $5'-$ adenosine monophosphate

(cyclic AMP, cAMP) inside the cell (Figure 12). It is this cyclic AMP that is the intracellular hormonal mediator, which brings about specific cellular changes (Figure 13). Cyclic AMP is sometimes referred to as a secondary chemical messenger, the first messenger being the stimulating hormone. Cyclic AMP is a nucleotide and is called a second messenger because it transmits and amplifies within the cell, the chemical signals which are delivered by the hormones that are circulating throughout the bloodstream. These hormones are of course the first messengers. The cyclic AMP mechanism is the mode used by many hormones to stimulate their target tissue. Some of these hormones include: (1) catecholamines (epinephrine and norepinephrine), (2) thyroid-stimulating hormone (thyrotropin, TSH), (3) parathyroid hormone (parathormone, PTH), (4) luteinizing hormone (LH), (5) follicle-stimulating hormone (FSH), (6) adrenocorticotropic hormone (adrenocorticotropin, corticotropin, ACTH), (7), antidiuretic hormone (vasopressin, ADH), and (8) the hypothalamic releasing factors (hormones) that control secretion of most of the anterior pituitary hormones.

Another intracellular mediator or secondary messenger is cyclic guanosine monophosphate (cGMP) which is also a cyclic nucleotide, similar to cyclic AMP. The only difference is that it contains the base guanine rather than adenine. It is known to play a role in specific regulatory mechanisms of the body. While cAMP and cGMP are activated in a similar manner, they differ in the intracellular reactions which they mediate. Hence two separate second messenger control mechanisms can operate simultaneously in the same cell yet function independently. In summary, both cyclic AMP and cyclic GMP play a key role in the biochemical actions of a number of hormones.

There are other types of intracellular hormonal

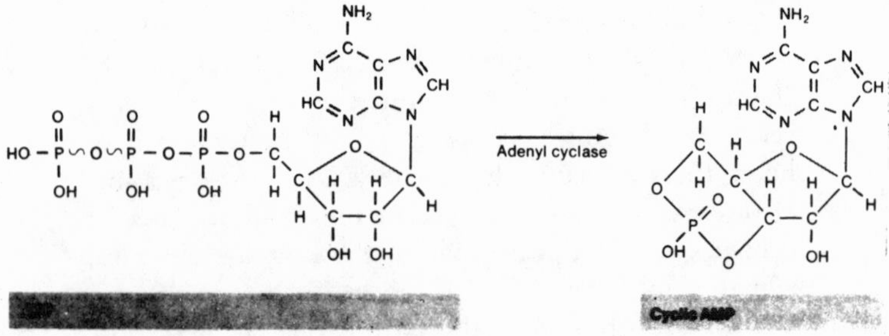

Figure 12
The formation of cyclic AMP from ATP.

mediators. A group of lipid compounds, derivatives
of fatty acids, ubiquitously present throughout the
body, called the prostaglandins, may function as such
hormonal mediators. These substances have been
postulated to mediate several hundreds of various cellular control functions.

(2) Another mechanism of hormonal action involves
hormones entering the cell directly, passing through
the cell membrane, and then binding to cytoplasmic
receptors. Hormone receptor binding is then followed
by an activation process and translocation to the
nucleus where the activated receptors bind to DNA
and nuclear proteins. This is followed by the production of specific RNA molecules. The RNA then dif-
fuses out of the nucleus and into the cytoplasm where
it stimulates the synthesis of specific proteins. These
proteins then function as carrier proteins to increase
specific activities of the cells which result in specific
physiological responses (Figure 14). For example, in
the presence of the hormone aldosterone, protein enzymes are formed in the renal tubules which results in
sodium reabsorption and potassium secretion. There

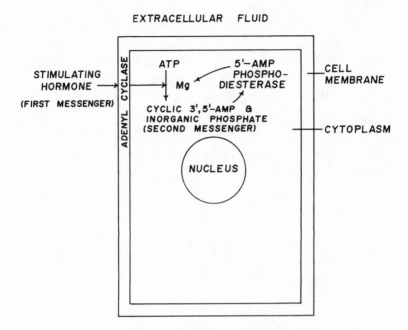

Figure 13
Mechanism of action of hormones through activation of cAMP.

is a characteristic delay of 45 minutes to several hours or days for full activity of this hormone to be realized. This is to be contrasted with the peptide-derived hormones whose cellular effects are seen quite rapidly. This mechanism of activated receptor binding to the gene material of the nucleus is the method by which the steroid hormones act to initiate protein production in their target cells, thereby activating certain cellular functions.

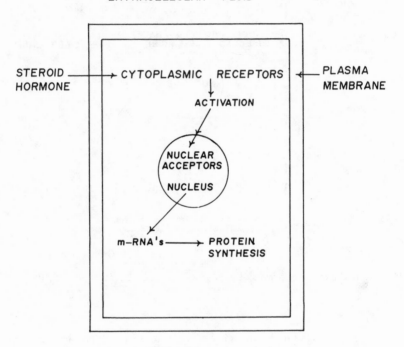

Figure 14
Mechanism of action of steroid hormones.

CHAPTER 5

Pituitary Gland

The pituitary gland is also known as the hypophysis. It is a small gland about 1 cm (0.4 inch) in diameter and approximately 0.5 to 1 gram in weight. It is located at the base of the brain (Figure 4) and is attached to the hypothalamus by the pituitary or hypophyseal stalk.

The gland is seen to be made up of two distinct portions, namely the anterior pituitary (adenohypophysis) and the posterior pituitary (neurohypophysis). Between these two zones is the pars intermedia, a small and relatively avascular zone. This zone is quite small or almost absent in humans, while it is much larger and plays a greater functional role in some lower animals.

The anterior lobe of the pituitary secretes six important hormones and several less important ones. The most important hormones include growth hormone (GH), adrenocorticotropic hormone (ACTH), thyroid-stimulating hormone (TSH), follicle-stimulating hormone (FSH), luteinizing hormone (LH), and prolactin (P).

The way in which the major anterior pituitary hormones exert their physiological effects is to stimulate various target glands throughout the body. The glands influenced include the thyroid, adrenal cortex, the gonads (i.e., the testes and ovaries and mammary glands). Growth hormone is the exception and exerts its influence on all the tissues of the body that are capable of growth. Generally speaking, the anterior pituitary hormones play a part in controlling metabolic activities of the body. GH functions to control the growth of the organism as a whole. It influences the metabolic activities of many cells throughout the body and plays a major role in protein formation. ACTH regulates the secretion of hormones of the adrenal cortex, which in turn influences the metabolism of proteins, glucose, and fats. TSH regulates the secretion of hormones of the thyroid gland. These hormones control the rate of metabolism and the rate of growth of the reproductive organs. Prolactin plays a role in the development of the mammary glands and production of milk.

It is known that upon elicitation of the stress response, heightened physiological activity occurs. This in turn strongly influences metabolic activity. Since metabolic activity is directly related to anterior pituitary function, it is easy to see how these anterior pituitary hormones are implicated in the whole stress phenomenon.

PITUITARY GLAND AND ITS RELATIONSHIP TO THE HYPOTHALAMUS

Anterior Pituitary

Almost all of the pituitary hormonal secretions are controlled by the brain: in particular, the hypothalamus. Hormonal or nervous signals from the hypothalamus regulate hormonal secretions from the pituitary gland. The anterior portion of the pituitary is controlled by tropic hormones called hypothalamic releasing and inhibiting hormones, or factors which are secreted by specialized neurons within the hypothalamus itself. These tropic hormones then travel through minute blood vessels called hypothalamic-hypophyseal portal vessels, that lead from the hypothalamus to the anterior pituitary. These releasing or tropic hormones act on the anterior pituitary glandular cells, thereby controlling their secretions.

Hypothalamic Releasing Hormones

At the present time, it is thought that most of the hypothalamic hormones are released at nerve endings located in the median eminence, before they are conducted through the portal vessels to the anterior pituitary (Figure 15).

Each hypothalamic releasing hormone controls the secretion of a particular anterior pituitary hormone. Also, hypothalamic inhibiting hormones exist for some anterior pituitary hormones. For example, the anterior pituitary hormone, prolactin, is regulated more by a hypothalamic inhibiting hormone (PIH) than by a releasing hormone (PRH). The major hypothalamic releasing and inhibiting hormones are:

(1) Corticotropin releasing hormone (CRH) which regulates the secretion of anterior pituitary adrenocorticotropin (ACTH),

(2) Growth hormone releasing hormone (GHRH) which regulates the secretion of anterior pituitary growth hormone (GH) and growth hormone inhibiting hormone (GHIH) also known as somatostatin, which inhibits the release of growth hormone,

(3) Thyroid-stimulating hormone releasing hormone (TRH) which regulates the release of thyrotropin also known as thyroid stimulating hormone (TSH) by the anterior pituitary,

(4) Luteinizing hormone releasing hormone (LHRH) or gonadotropin releasing hormone (GnRH) which regulates anterior pituitary release of both luteinizing hormone (LH) and follicle-stimulating hormone (FSH), and

(5) Prolactin releasing hormone (PRH) and prolactin inhibiting hormone (PIH) which regulates the stimulation and inhibition of secretion of prolactin by the anterior pituitary.

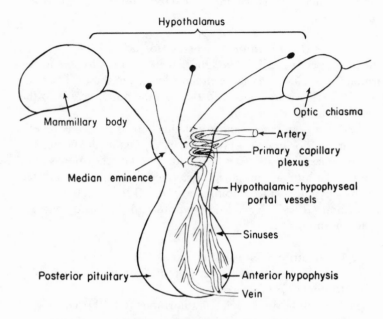

Figure 15
Hypothalamic control of the anterior pituitary. The hypothalamic-hypo-
physial portal system. Adapted from A.C. Guyton, *Textbook of Medical
Physiology*, (6th ed.). Philadelphia: W.B. Saunders Co., 1981, p. 921.

Posterior Pituitary

In the posterior pituitary, there are great numbers of terminal
nerve endings, which belong to nerve tracts that originate in the
regions of the hypothalamus called the supraoptic nuclei and
paraventricular nuclei. The hypophyseal or pituitary stalk is the
means whereby these nerve tracts pass from the hypothalamus to
the pituitary (Figure 16). It is believed that two hormones are
synthesized in the nerve cell bodies of these two regions of the
hypothalamus and are transported by means of carrier proteins

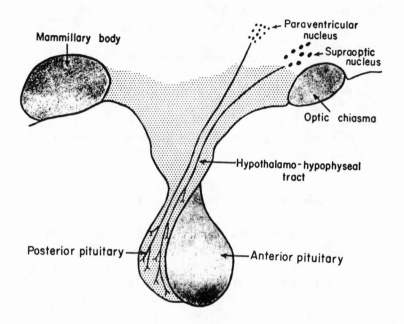

Figure 16
Hypothalamic control of the posterior pituitary. The hypothalamic-hypophysial neuronal tracts. Adapted from A.C. Guyton, *Textbook of Medical Physiology*, (6th ed.). Philadelphia: W.B. Saunders Co., 1981, p. 927.

(neurophysins) to the terminal nerve endings, which lie in the posterior pituitary. From the time of synthesis to the time of hormonal release by the posterior pituitary, several days may elapse.

The posterior pituitary secretes two important hormones, namely antidiuretic hormone, ADH (vasopressin), which is formed primarily in the supraoptic nuclei, the oxytocin, formed principally in the paraventricular nuclei.

ADH is a hormone that plays a role in fluid balance and regulates the rate of urinary water excretion. Scientific data suggest that ADH secretion is affected by stress. Oxytocin, on the other hand, helps in the delivery of milk from the milk glands and may play a role in the delivery process at the end of gestation. The stress of labor has been shown to influence oxytocin secretion.

Pars Intermedia

The pituitary is also composed of a small segment called the Pars Intermedia. This section of the pituitary gland secretes a hormone called Melanocyte-Stimulating hormone (MSH). Its physiological effect in humans appears to be insignificant and, as yet, its role remains to be elucidated.

IMPLICATION FOR THE STRESS RESPONSE

The hypothalamus itself is the recipient of information through signal transmission from nearly all parts of the nervous system. It collects information concerned with the well-being of the organism. For example, information concerned with body temperature, concentrations of nutrients, electrolytes, and various hormones, is collected by the hypothalamus. Also when a subject experiences an exciting or depressing thought, a portion of that signal is transmitted to the hypothalamus. Information on a person's emotional state is also recorded. So, depending on the signals received, various portions of the hypothalamus are excited or inhibited. This excitation or inhibition of various portions of the hypothalamus in turn influences hypothalamic control of pituitary gland secretions. Since the elicitation of the stress response is tied into the mental and emotional states of the individual, one can easily see how the immediate effects of this response could influence hypothalamic inputs, which in turn affect pituitary secretions.

ANTERIOR PITUITARY HORMONES

As mentioned previously, the anterior pituitary secretes a number of tropic hormones. We shall not take up a discussion of these hormones here, but will discuss them in the chapters that cover their respective target glands. Instead, we shall proceed with a discussion of growth hormone, since it has no specific target gland as its domain of influence, but instead exerts its effect on all the cells in the body.

Growth Hormone

Growth Hormone (GH), also known as somatotropic hormone (SH) or somatotropin, is secreted by the anterior pituitary gland, and stimulates the growth of body cells.

This hormone also has many metabolic effects. It enhances amino acid movement across cell membranes into cells, thereby causing an increase in the rate of cellular utilization of these substances. Increased rate of protein synthesis in all cells is the result. While protein breakdown is diminished by GH, almost all facets of cellular amino acid uptake and protein synthesis are stimulated.

Decreased rate of cellular carbohydrate utilization is also the result of GH secretion. In other words, the rate which glucose is employed by all the cells throughout the body is decreased. The net effect of GH on carbohydrate metabolism results in a reduction of cellular glucose uptake, a decrease in glucose utilization for energy, and an increase in glucose stores in the cell in the form of glycogen deposits. The effect here is that GH can lead to a rise in blood sugar levels. This increase in blood sugar levels can in turn stimulate the beta cells of the pancreatic islets of Langerhans to secrete extra insulin. There is also a further mild stimulatory effect of GH on the beta cells directly. Both of these effects can summate to cause an overstimulation of insulin secrtion. This can result in a disease called diabetes mellitus. Growth hormone is therefore a potential diabetogenic agent.

On the other hand, under the influence of this hormone, cells are stimulated to increase the rate of fat utilization for energy. In essence, the adipose tissues of the body are stimulated to convert their reserves into fatty acids (lipolysis), which result in an elevation of the circulating levels of free fatty acids. Hence, GH results in the increased utilization of fats for energy in place of both carbohydrates and proteins. It must be stated that the GH stimulation of fatty acid utilization takes hours to occur, whereas the synthesis of cellular proteins under growth hormone occurs quite rapidly.

In summary, the metabolic effects of GH include: (1) enhancement of body protein, (2) enhancement in the utilization of fat reserves, and (3) carbohydrate conservation. The exact mechanism whereby GH exerts these physiological effects has not been clearly elucidated.

Growth hormone secretion is influenced by various factors. Its release is mainly stimulated by GHRH from the hypothalamus. Also, it has been observed that the nutritional state of the individual influences GH activity. It appears that the hypothalamus is a good sensor of blood nutrient concentrations and secretes GHRH accordingly. For example, GH is secreted more during states of protein deficiency and during conditions of abnormally low blood glucose levels. Also GHIH (somatostatin) plays a minor role in growth hormone secretion. It must be stated that the delta cells of the islets of Langerhans also secrete somatostatin. Somatostatin is known to inhibit insulin and glucagon secretion by the islets of Langerhans. Hence this hormone may have many functions in several hormonal processes (Guyton, 1981).

Growth Hormone also has an effect on many of the electrolytes found in the body. One can observe retention of sodium, potassium, phosphate, and calcium in the body, as a result of GH influence.

There are several conditions which develop as a result of undersecretion or oversecretion of GH, during both childhood and adulthood. Abnormal conditions such as dwarfism, giantism, and acromegaly can occur in such cases. However, it is not the purpose of this text to discuss such abnormalities. Rather, the purpose is to focus on those physiological effects of growth hormone secretion that are concerned with normal nutrient levels, which contribute to homeostasis and its alteration during the stress response.

Growth Hormone and Stress

There is evidence that besides regulation of GH secretion by the hypothalamic releasing hormones, the central nervous system may also function in controlling the release of GH.

In humans, the stress of surgery has been observed to increase GH levels in the bloodstream. The stress of rising out of bed in the morning, which of course can be experienced by many individuals as very stressful, also results in an increase in the secretion of GH. Fasting in humans results in hypoglycemia and this in turn can trigger an increase in the secretion of GH. Hyperglycemia on the other hand inhibits GH secretion.

It might be stated that the elicitation of the stress response may result in altered levels of amino acids, glucose, and fatty acids in the circulation. Any of the metabolites or combinations of these metabolites may be changed from normal levels as a result of the stress response. The plasma levels of these three metabolites may very well be the dominant regulator of GH secretion. Therefore, whatever the prevailing circulatory levels of these metabolites are, as a result of the elicitation of the stress response, will determine whether GH secretion is enhanced or depressed.

With regard to animal experiments, in the laboratory rat the stress of fasting does not result in an increase in GH secretion. Perhaps this is so because the rat may possess a different neuroendocrine and neurochemical response pattern when exposed to various types of stressors. A study exposing laboratory rats to cold stress and the stress of forced immobilization was reported by Lenox et al. (1980). These researchers reported an elevation in plasma corticosterone (the major glucocorticoid in the rat), concomitant with a decrease in plasma GH in the laboratory animals exposed to stressors. Other studies involving rats, which demonstrate a decrease in GH, have been reported in the literature by Brown and Martin (1974), Henkin and Knigge (1963), and Kokka et al. (1972). On the other hand, studies in rhesus and squirrel monkeys have demonstrated a high responsivity to GH (Brown et al., 1971; Mason et al., 1968; and Meyer et al., 1967).

As far as human responsivity to GH secretion during psychological stress is concerned, several investigations are currently underway. Some of the research available points to the fact that with various psychological stimuli, GH levels become elevated, particularly in those subjects who can be categorized as most anxious (Schalach, 1967).

Miyabo et al. (1975) report a study concerned with the induction

of psychological stress in control and neurotic subjects. The results
of their study show that the GH and cortisol levels changed mini-
mally in normal subjects, indicating the presence of an effective
psychoneuroendocrine coping mechanism. In neurotic subjects,
GH and cortisol levels were elevated and greater than the control
group. Hence in the neurotic group, these researchers claim that the
psychoneuroendocrine homeostasis was not very well maintained.
They observed a negative correlation between GH and cortisol in
the neurotic subjects.

Summary

Growth hormone secretion tends to increase in humans as a result of the elicitation of the stress response. For example, the stress
of surgery, electroshock therapy, physical exercise, and other physical stimuli all enhance GH secretion. Psychogenic stimuli, such as
the anticipation of strenuous and exhausting exercise, and performance tests which are anxiety evoking, all enhance GH secretion.
The responses of GH secretion to stress do not occur as frequently
as the cortisol responses. Increases in GH secretion are usually
found in subjects who already have elevated cortisol levels.

The role of GH as a result of the stress response may be similar to
that of glucagon, namely to stimulate the uptake of amino acids by
cells and to mobilize the energy resources of the body.

It might be added that there are other hormones which also play a
role in influencing the secretion of GH. For example, the presence
of the thyroid hormone, thyroxine, is necessary for both the synthesis and secretion of GH. The hormones, glucagon, estrogen, and
epinephrine enhance the secretion of GH, while excessive amounts
of cortisol depresses its secretion. It might be stated that as a result
of the elicitation of the stress response, GH secretion may also be
influenced by the prevailing circulating levels of these respective
hormones.

PARS INTERMEDIA HORMONES

Melanocyte Stimulating Hormone

The pars intermedia of the pituitary gland manufactures minute amounts of a hormone called melanocyte stimulating hormone (MSH). Since this hormone comes from the intermediate lobe of the pituitary, MSH is also referred to as Intermedin. This hormone plays a role in influencing the pigment cells of the skin (melanophores) to expand and increase the synthesis of melanin (melanogenesis). Melanin darkens the skin, and administering large doses of MSH promotes in both humans and animals, a pronounced darkening of the skin. Physiologically, this hormone appears to have much more heightened activity in the lower animal kingdom than in the human. It the lower animal kingdom, this darkening of the skin, which acts to camouflage the animal with its ambient environment, offers an important protective device. However, in the human, insignificant amounts of MSH are produced, and its physiological effects remain unknown. Adrenocorticotropin hormone (ACTH) possesses a function in humans which is similar to MSH. MSH secretion, like the other anterior pituitary hormones, is controlled by hypothalamic releasing hormones, namely MSHRH and MSHIH. MSHIH is probably the most important controller of MSH release, since the main hypothalamic effect seems to be one of tonic inhibition of MSH secretion by the pars intermedia of the anterior pituitary. This lends itself to further clarification.

Today it is recognized that at least two distinct forms of MSH exist which are known as α-MSH and β-MSH. These hormones are both small polypeptides and contain within their amino acid chains a heptapeptide sequence which is also present in adrenocorticotropin (ACTH) and the lipotropins (LPH). The most potent mammalian melanocyte stimulating peptide known is α-MSH, although in humans β-MSH accounts for almost all of the plasma MSH activity. Also present in the intermediate lobe of the pituitary are small amounts of ACTH (Kraicer et al., 1973; Kraicer & Morris, 1976a,b), which is often referred to as (PI) ACTH to distinguish it from the ACTH that is secreted by the anterior pituitary.

In humans, factors which influence ACTH secretion seem to influence MSH secretion. Thus it appears that MSH secretion parallels that of ACTH. However, both ACTH and MSH can be secreted independently, both in humans and in experimental animals.

Melanocyte Stimulating Hormone and Stress

Factors which increase ACTH secretion, such as stress, also increase MSH secretion. Both hormones exhibit a diurnal rhythm.

In humans, it has been suggested that MSH is secreted during Hypoadrenalism (Sulman, 1956; Lerner, 1961; and Abe et al., 1976b). In the rat, however, MSH secretion does not seem to be affected by adrenal function. Several researchers report that it is secreted in higher amounts in the rat during stress (Thody et al., 1975b; and Kastin et al., 1969).

Kraicer et al. (1977) studied the effects of (PI) ACTH and α-MSH and pars distalis ACTH (anterior pituitary) concentration during some stress experiments. Stresses, such as adrenalectomy, gonadectomy, and neurotropic (noise) stress were induced in experimental laboratory rats. These researchers found that: (1) ACTH release following adrenalectomy was unaccompanied by changes in (PI) ACTH and MSH content: (2) the feedback-induced gonadotropin increased secretion following gonadectomy was associated with significant changes in PI ACTH and MSH contents: and (3) the stress of noise resulted in significant increases in (PI) ACTH and MSH. These researchers found a positive correlation between (PI) ACTH and MSH contents and concluded that (PI) ACTH and MSH secretions are altered in response to change in gonadotropin secretion and neurotropic stressors. This study might be compared with the results of other similar studies which indicate stimulatory or inhibitory effects on MSH secretion as a reuslt of sex differentiation (Coyne & Kitay, 1969; Taleisnik & Tomats, 1969).

There are a few studies which report no effect on MSH secretion in the presence of a neurogenic stressor (Kastin et al., 1967; and

Brown et al., 1974). However, in one particular study, an increase in plasma MSH was found after the stress of foot shock (Sandman et al., 1973).

Summary

These studies and others not discussed here open the way for continuous investigations into the relative roles of the pars inter-media and anterior pituitary in adrenal cortical function. The role of (PI) ACTH in hypothalamic-pituitary-adrenal cortical function remains to be elucidated. Also yet to be clarified is the physiological significance of any change in MSH activity as it relates to the stress response.

It might be added here that hypothalamic catecholamines appear to have an important role in regulating the secretion of MSH. While the catecholamines may influence the secretion of hypo-thalamic MSHIH through neurotransmitter activity, they may also directly influence pituitary MSH secretion. It is not clear at this point whether this has any implication for the stress response.

POSTERIOR PITUITARY HORMONES

Antidiuretic hormone (ADH) and oxytocin are two hormones that are released from nerve endings and absorbed into adjacent capillaries when nerve signals are conducted down the nerve fiber of the posterior pituitary. These hormones are polypeptides consist-ing of eight amino acids bonded together. The molecules of both substances are similar with the exception of the presence of two amino acids.

Oxytocin

Oxytocin plays a role in the process of lactation and in the labor process. During the process of lactation, this hormone causes milk to be released from the alveoli and into the ducts of the mammary gland. In this way, the baby can obtain it by suckling. It is believed that suckling causes signals to be transmitted via sensory nerves that lead to the hypothalamus. The hypothalamus then signals the posterior pituitary to release oxytocin, which is then carried through the circulatory system where it reaches the mammary glands and causes the contraction of myoepithelial cells.

Oxytocin is a hormone that is also released toward the end of pregnancy. It stimulates uterine contractions and therefore plays a role in the stress of labor. The mechanism of hormone action is not clear but it is thought that the stretching of uterine tissues may result in nerve signal transmission to the hypothalamus, which in turn relays information to the posterior pituitary to release oxytocin. ADH also stimulates the pregnant uterus but its effect is very small. Also, oxytocin can excite other smooth muscles in the body to contract.

Antidiuretic Hormone

A substance that enhances the rate of urine formation is called a diuretic. An antidiuretic then is a substance that depresses urine formation. ADH is just such a substance, and it performs its antidiuretic activity by acting directly on the kidney, to regulate its urine output. In particular, the water permeability of the collecting ducts in the terminal portion of the nephrons changes under the influence of ADH. Therefore, ADH has an important function in the regulation of the water content of body fluid compartments. It only takes a very small amount of ADH in the bloodstream to produce an antidiuresis. ADH secretion is under hypothalamic control. What appears to happen is that certain neurons in this part of the brain are sensitive to changes in the osmolality of the blood. These neurons are referred to as osmoreceptors. For example, when a person is sweating and undergoes a large water loss, the blood becomes more concentrated. This change in the blood is sensed by the osmoreceptors, and the posterior pituitary is then signalled to release ADH. The immediate effect of ADH on the kidneys is an increase in fluid reabsorption due to permeability changes in the terminal portion of the nephrons. This results in less urine production and therefore water conservation. On the other hand, when a person drinks water in excess, thereby diluting the body fluids, ADH release is inhibited. In this case, urine flow is enhanced and a more dilute urine is excreted by the kidneys. The water concentration in the body fluids then returns to normal. It is known that 95 percent of the total osmotic pressure of the extracellular body fluids is determined by sodium. Since ADH secretion is very sensitive to the osmolality of the blood, we find ADH to be a very potent agent in controlling the sodium ion concentration of the body fluids. Besides a rise in plasma osmolality, a fall in plasma volume such as occurs in hemorrhage also increases ADH secretion. This increase is mediated through vascular receptors located in the atria of the heart and in the carotid sinuses. In this case, it is the vagus nerve that sends signals to the appropriate brain centers to signal the release of ADH.

Also, ADH, in mid to high concentrations, has a very potent arteriolar vasoconstrictor effect. Because of this effect, ADH is sometimes referred to as vasopressin. It was thought that the concentrations of ADH that are normally found in the blood are too small to result in any significant pressor effect. However, recent work has shown that when arterial pressure is lowered, ADH is subsequently secreted in amounts to elevate the pressure to at least 75 percent of its original value (Guyton, 1981). It is indicated now that ADH may play a much greater role in arterial pressure homeostasis than was previously thought.

It might be added here that both norepinephrine and the prostaglandins may exert an inhibitory influence on the renal action of ADH. The mechanisms involved are not clear, although it is thought that the prostaglandins may exert their influence on ADH by inhibiting the formation of cAMP, the intracellular mediator by which ADH mediates its physiological effects. It is interesting to note that norepinephrine, on the other hand, exerts an inhibitory action only in the presence of cortisol (Levi et al., 1973).

Antidiuretic Hormone and Stress

There are several factors, other than the changes in osmolality or plasma volume described above, that influence ADH secretion and results in an increase in its production. These include pharmacological interventions such as tranquilizers, some anesthetics, nicotine and morphine, and conditions of stress imposed upon the body such as trauma, pain, and anxiety. One can witness pronounced water retention in the body in the presence of these factors. It might be added that nausea also strongly influences the secretion of ADH.

The implication for the involvement of ADH in the stress response is evident. For example, in many stress-induced emotional states, water accumulation in the body frequently occurs. Afterwards, when such a state has subsided, a diuresis ensues. Another very popular stress reactive behavior is the drinking of alcohol. Alcoholic beverages, which contain ethyl alcohol, appear to inhibit ADH release. Therefore, subsequent to alcoholic intake, large amounts of urine are generally formed. Any body fluids lost from such a condition are later replaced. Alcohol may also cause the different arterioles of the kidney nephrons to dilate. This helps to enhance the diuretic state. Let us now consider some recent research involving stressful stimuli and ADH secretion.

The complex stress of surgery has been studied with regard to circulating levels of ADH (Moran & Zimmermann, 1967). In a patient undergoing a gastrectomy, these researchers have investigated preoperative and postoperative levels of circulating ADH. They found preoperative ADH levels to be increased, probably due to the anxiety of surgery. Postoperatively, ADH levels remained elevated until the fifth day. These authors also performed a similar experiment in the dog and found a comparable response in ADH levels.

In a study involving human subjects as described by Segar and Moore (1968), cold stress resulted in decreased levels of ADH accompanied by a diuresis. Subsequent elevations in temperature caused ADH levels to rise. These results can be explained by the activity of the volume receptors mentioned previously. During cold stress, peripheral vasoconstriction occurs and blood volume is confined to a smaller space. This in turn could cause the left atrial pressure to increase, with a resultant inhibition of ADH secretion. On the other hand, increased temperature results in a peripheral vasodilation. This is followed by a decrease in left atrial pressure with a resultant stimulation of ADH secretion.

The effects of anesthesia on ADH have been discussed at length by Philbin et al. (1977) and Philbin and Coggins (1978). These researchers found increased levels of ADH in human subjects. This would suggest that the effect of anesthesia on ADH levels may be due to the various hemodynamic changes accompanying anesthesia and not to the anesthetic itself. This hemodynamic change would necessarily precipitate decreased urine flow rates. In other words, if a decrease in urine flow is observed, then the primary stimulus is the hemodynamic effects of the anesthetic and the secondary stimulus is a release in ADH.

Several researchers have studied the interactions of ADH and cortisol. McCann et al. (1966) present evidence that vasopressin may play a small role in the adrenal cortical response to stress. Wiley et al. (1974), in their work with rats, found that vasopressin-deficient rats had a lower than normal plasma corticosterone concentration during stress, and this was at least partially due to the relative insensitivity of the adrenal glands to ACTH. It must be noted that in the rat, corticosterone is the major glucocorticoid. These researchers concluded that the presence of vasopressin in the internal environment during early life may influence the sensitivity of the adrenal glands.

With regard to human research, arginine vasopressin, AVP, the naturally occurring antidiuretic hormone in humans, has been shown to increase plasma ACTH, cortisol, and growth hormone in normal subjects (Staub et al., 1973; Gwinup et al., 1967; and Czarny et al., 1968). Whether there is a physiological role of ADH in the control of ACTH (or its releasing factor) remains to be determined.

An interesting study relating to factors which elevate AVP levels in the human neonate, is described by De Vane and Porter (1980). These researchers studied the conditions in newborn humans which affect increased levels of plasma concentrations of AVP. In particular, the levels of plasma AVP were studied in terms of fetal stress and complications of pregnancy. These authors studied the plasma

from both arterial and venous umbilical cord blood of infants immediately before and after delivery. Three types of delivery conditions were investigated: vaginal delivery, and cesarean section
before and after the onset of labor. Also, these groups were further
considered in terms of the status of the neonate during pregnancy,
labor, and at the time of delivery. The infants were considered
non-stressed if no intrapartum complications were present. On the
other hand, any abnormal cardiac rhythms or the presence of
meconium in the amniotic fluid were used as indices of fetal stress.
In their studies, these researchers found a significant increase in
AVP levels of cord plasma from infants who had been stressed, as
compared to infants who were not stressed, during the conditions
of pregnancy and labor. This was also seen during vaginal or cesarean section delivery and during or prior to labor. They found that
in stressed infants, the levels of AVP in cord plasma were often 10
to 20 times that found in nonstressed infants. These studies suggest
a direct relationship between stress and the high release of AVP by
the human fetus. Also, these studies show that the highest levels of
AVP in fetal cord plasma occurred in those infants who experienced
fetal bradycardia and meconium in the amniotic fluid. They found
that if meconium were present in the amniotic fluid, invariably this
would be accompanied by high levels of AVP in cord plasma.
These authors concluded that in human newborns, umbilical cord
plasma levels of AVP is a strong indicator of fetal stress. Indeed, the
passage of meconium into the amniotic fluid may be correlated
with the release of AVP during stress, since AVP is easily cleared
by the placenta.

These findings in the newborn are comparable to that observed
in the fetal lamb. Stressful conditions imposed upon the lamb fetus
resulted in significant levels of AVP (Daniel et al., 1978; Alexander
et al., 1972, 1974, 1976; and Weitzman et al., 1978). However,
Stark et al. (1979) report high levels of AVP only after the onset of
labor in the fetal lamb. With regard to human neonates, Hoppenstein et al. (1968) observed AVP levels to be higher in infants after
normal vaginal delivery, as compared to AVP levels found in the
systemic plasma of older infants. Chard et al. (1971) found high
concentrations of AVP in umbilical cord blood after spontaneous

delivery. These studies clearly show that higher levels of AVP in umbilical cord plasma, both in human and lamb neonates, appear to be linked to situations of fetal stress.

Summary

From the above discussion, it can be seen that in addition to the physiological changes noted in plasma osmolality and plasma volume, various environmental and psychogenic stimuli influence ADH secretion. These stimuli do not seem to operate in a negative feedback control system for ADH, but all of these stimuli probably act on the higher regions of the central nervous system encompassing extrahypothalamic as well as hypothalamic brain structures. The influence of higher neural centers on ADH secretion can be demonstrated by the experimental induction of diuresis or antidiuresis through psychogenic conditioning in both humans and dogs. Other brain structures involved in affecting ADH secretion include the emotional brain and the reticular activating system.

CHAPTER 6

Adrenal Gland

The adrenal glands are paired organs situated at the top of each kidney. They are composed of two parts, namely the cortex and the medulla (Figure 17). The adrenal cortex and medulla, which secrete different types of hormones, are controlled by different mechanisms. It can be said that, functionally, the adrenal gland behaves as two separate and distinct endocrine glands combined into one. Surrounded by the outer cortex, the adrenal medulla secretes two important catecholamines: the amine hormones, norepinephrine and epinephrine. The adrenal cortex on the other hand secretes a number of steroid hormones.

ADRENAL MEDULLA

The fibers of the sympathetic nervous system control the secretion of the adrenal medulla. These fibers terminate on medullary tissue without a synapse. Hence, the adrenal medullary response is quite rapid.

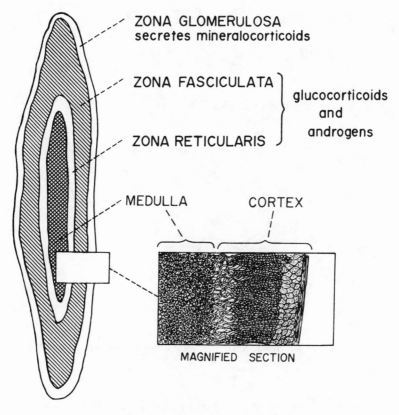

Figure 17
Secretion of adrenocortical hormones by the different zones of the adrenal cortex. Illustration of the anatomical zones of the adrenal cortex, and their secretions. The adrenal medulla is also shown. Adapted from A.C. Guyton, *Textbook of Medical Physiology*, (6th ed.). Philadelphia: W.B. Saunders Co., 1981, p. 953.

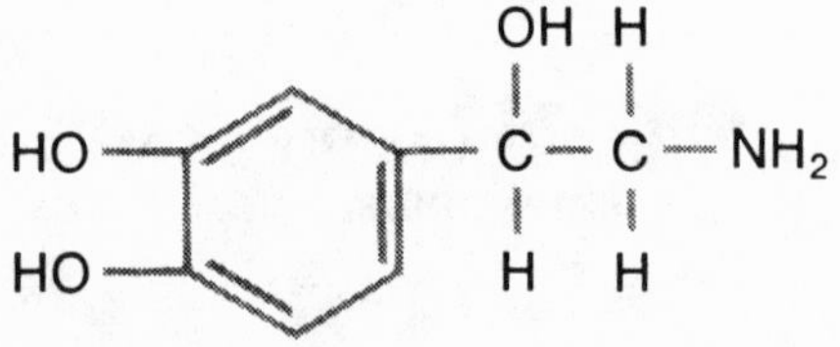

Norepinephrine

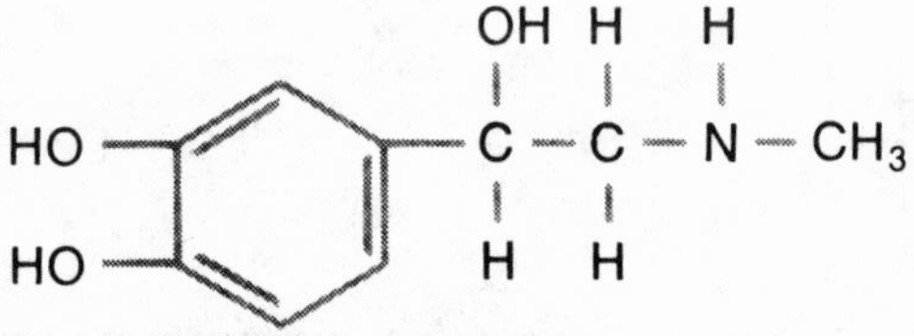

Epinephrine

Figure 18

The structures of the adrenal medullary hormones, epinephrine and norepinephrine.

The two active hormones secreted by the medulla are norepinephrine (noradrenaline) and epinephrine (adrenaline) (Figure 18). As can be seen from the figure, both of these substances have similar structures. Their functions are also similar. These hormones cause similar physiological effects on the body as direct stimulation of the sympathetic nervous system. Hence, they are referred to as "sympathomimetic" substances. However, the effects of these hormones last about 10 times as long as sympathetic activity because these hormones are removed from the circulation rather slowly.

The secretion of the adrenal medulla is approximately 80 percent

epinephrine and 20 percent norepinephrine. Some of
ical effects of these hormones include an increase in l
heart rate, respiration, blood sugar levels, and a dep...
tract activity. These effects are reminiscent of those described as
part of the physiological changes which occur as a result of sympathetic nervous system activation during the elicitation of the stress
response.

PHYSIOLOGICAL EFFECTS OF EPINEPHRINE AND
NOREPINEPHRINE

Central Nervous System

Epinephrine enhances anxiety by inducing arousal of the organism. This response is mediated through activation of portions of
the reticular formation. Norepinephrine is not as potent in producing this effect.

Respiratory System

Both epinephrine and norepinephrine cause the bronchi and
bronchioles to dilate and stimulate breathing. However, norepinephrine is not as potent as epinephrine in this regard.

Gastrointestinal System

Epinephrine and norepinephrine are effective in decreasing the
tone of the smooth muscles of the gastrointestinal tract (inhibits
peristaltic movement). The muscular contraction of the stomach is
also inhibited. Both catecholamines are effective in causing contraction of the pyloric sphincter. The overall effect is the slowing down
of digestion.

Circulatory System

The effects of the catecholamines on the circulatory system are
influenced mainly by epinephrine. Epinephrine causes a lowering

of the eosinophil count in the blood. Epinephrine decreases the coagulation time of the blood and aids in increasing the number of red blood cells. Cortisol has been known to aid epinephrine in lowering the eosinophil count. It may be that enhanced movement of fluids from the blood compartment into the intercellular fluid spaces, resulting in hemoconcentration, may account for the above-described changes induced by epinephrine.

In the cardiovascular system, both epinephrine and norepinephrine will increase heart rate (positive chronotropic effect), and the force of contraction of the muscles of the heart (positive inotropic effect). Epinephrine and norepinephrine have also been shown to constrict the blood vessels of the periphery (skin) and splanchnic bed. In the blood vessels of skeletal muscles, epinephrine has a dilation effect, whereas norepinephrine will cause these vessels to constrict.

Both epinephrine and norepinephrine differ in their effects on blood pressure. Norepinephrine increases overall peripheral resistance because of its much more general vasoconstrictor effect in the body. This is due to its influence on the skeletal muscle vasculature. Also, since the stroke volume of the heart (the amount of blood ejected from the ventricle per beat) is elevated, the blood pressure (both systolic and diastolic) are raised. Hence, the result is an increase in mean arterial pressure. Epinephrine, on the other hand, may or may not change the mean arterial pressure. This is because epinephrine generally raises systolic pressure while exerting little if any effect on diastolic pressure. This effect is related to the vasodilation which occurs in skeletal muscle and vasoconstriction which occurs in the periphery and splanchnic region. Hence, this dual effect may result in an overall decrease in peripheral resistance. Additionally, since stroke volume is elevated, diastolic pressure may fall slightly.

In regard to metabolism, epinephrine has been shown to increase the basal metabolic rate and is therefore considered to be calorigenic (increases total oxygen consumption). Epinephrine also acts on both the liver and the pancreas. In the liver, it enhances glycogenolysis and gluconeogenesis. In the pancreas, both epinephrine and norepinephrine can inhibit the glucose-induced secretion of insulin.

These effects lead to elevated levels of glucose. Because of this effect, epinephrine is considered a potent hyperglycemic agent. Epinephrine has also been shown to stimulate glycogenolysis in skeletal muscles.

Additional Effects of the Catecholamines

Additional effects of the catecholamines include: Stimulation of salivary secretion and secretion of the lacrimal glands by epinephrine. Both epinephrine and norepinephrine stimulate sweating, and dilation of the pupils.

Many of the catecholamine effects are similar for both epinephrine and norepinephrine, but some differences exist. The major differences lie in the following;

(1) Epinephrine has a more pronounced effect on the heart than norepinephrine,

(2) Norepinephrine causes a much more potent vasoconstrictor effect on the blood vessels of muscles than epinephrine. The effect is quite pronounced since muscle vascularization represents a large portion of total body vasculature. Hence, as described previously, blood pressure and total peripheral resistance are greatly elevated by norepinephrine. Epinephrine raises blood pressure only to a lesser degree, and

(3) Epinephrine has a much greater influence on elevating metabolic rate than does norepinephrine. It is known that epinephrine can elevate metabolism by as much as 100 percent above normal. You can see that this is a way of enhancing hyperactivity of the whole body.

In summary, it is the impulse transmission along the sympathetic nervous system that influences the adrenal medulla to secrete its hormones. Generally speaking, these impulses take their origin in the hypothalamus in response to various types of stressful stimuli. Therefore it can be seen that the adrenal medullary hormones function together with the sympathetic nervous system to prepare the

heightened energy needed in eliciting the stress re-
at is commonly called the "fight or flight" response.
ribed, is the first of the neuroendocrine pathways or
axes which are activated upon elicitation of the stress response.

ADRENAL CORTEX

The adrenal cortex consists of three distinct zones, namely, an
outer zone called the zona glomerulosa, a center zone called the
zona fasciculata, and an inner zone called the zona reticularis.

The adrenal cortex secretes two major types of hormones,
namely, the mineralocorticoids and the glucocorticoids. The zona
glomerulosa produces the mineralocorticoids which play a role in
influencing the electrolytes of the extracellular fluids. The principal
mineralocorticoid is aldosterone. This zone seems to be controlled,
for the most part, by the renin–angiotensin system. The zona fasciculata produces the glucocorticoids which, as the name implies,
influences blood glucose levels. In addition to carbohydrate
metabolism, the glucocorticoids also influence protein and fat
metabolism. The major glucocorticoid is cortisol.

The adrenal cortex, in addition to secreting mineralocorticoids
and glucocorticoids, also secretes a small quantity of sex hormones.
The most important are the androgens which basically have the
same effects as testosterone, the prominent male sex hormone. In
normal situations, because of the small amounts of circulating androgens, the androgens are of relatively little importance. However, their influence becomes greatly magnified in certain abnormal
conditions of the adrenal cortex. The adrenal origin of the androgens is the zona reticularis. Both the zona fasciculata and zona
reticularis seem to be controlled by ACTH.

A large number of steroid hormones have been isolated from the
adrenal cortex, but two of these hormones, aldosterone and cortisol, play a major role in human and animal endocrinology (Figure
19). The adrenal steroids have also been shown to influence the
immune system of the body. The role played by cortisol on im-

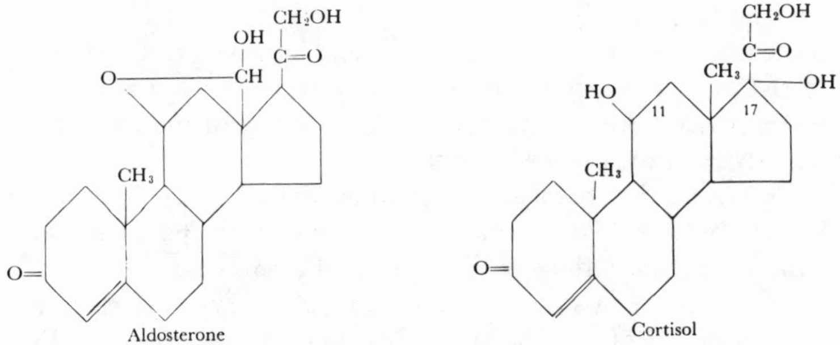

Figure 19
The two most important corticosteroids, aldosterone and cortisol.

muno-suppression will be discussed later in this chapter and in Chapter 12.

Mineralocorticoids

The major mineralocorticoid is aldosterone, and its primary function is to regulate the reabsorption of sodium from the glomerular filtrate, gastric juice, sweat, and saliva, in order to keep sodium at normal levels in the blood. Any slight increase in aldosterone secretion will increase the sodium levels in the blood. However, when the blood level of aldosterone increases, the result is an increase in the extracellular sodium concentration. Under normal circumstances, this situation does not occur since the thirst mechanism is activated concomitant with the above. This results in the drinking of water which will dilute the body fluids, thereby decreasing the extracellular sodium concentration.

Aldosterone, while enhancing sodium reabsorption, also enhances potassium secretion by the distal and collecting tubules of the kidney. Under the influence of aldosterone, the kidneys excrete large amounts of potassium. This is the primary mechanism by which the body maintains the potassium concentration at normal levels in the blood.

The quantities of sodium, chloride, and bicarbonate in the blood are elevated under the influence of aldosterone. The net result is that mineralocorticoid activity markedly changes the amount of electrolytes in the extracellular fluid.

The factors that regulate aldosterone secretion include: state of the intravascular fluid volume, concentration of the potassium ions in the extracellular fluid compartment, the renin-angiotensin system, the amount of sodium in the body, the nervous system, and the adrenocorticotropic hormone (ACTH). The physiological effects of aldosterone are believed to be mediated through the nuclear transcription process (the synthesis of RNA from DNA template).

Aldosterone and Stress

An important stimulus for aldosterone secretion is a drop in plasma volume. This also acts as a stimulant for sympathetic nervous system activation. It is known that various anxiety states and trauma activate the sympathetic nervous system, as well as enhance aldosterone secretion. Hence, it appears as though, as a result of an anxiety state, input from the central nervous system will lead to parallel changes in both the sympathetic nervous system and aldosterone secretion. In addition to the above-mentioned physiological factors that determine aldosterone secretion, the central nervous system may play a distinct role.

During stress, an increase in aldosterone secretion leads to water retention. Since more sodium is reabsorbed into the circulation, more water must follow in order to maintain the osmotic pressure close to normal levels. As a result of stress, enhanced aldosterone secretion coupled with an increase in ADH secretion contributes toward increased water retention in the body. This typically is seen in various states of stress. It is also thought that the pineal gland may secrete a hormone which stimulates aldosterone secretion. This observation as it relates to the stress response must await further investigative work.

Both angiotensin II and the sympathetic nervous system may play a role in stimulating aldosterone secretion. The elicitation of the stress response results not only in a stimulation of the sympathetic nervous system, but also of the renin-angiotensin system. The secretion of renin enhances the secretion of angiotensin II, which in turn increases the secretion of aldosterone. Both hormones, angiotensin II and aldosterone, are generally elevated as a result of the stress response.

ACTH, at the levels in which it is found in the blood, does not have too much effect on aldosterone secretion. However, elevations in ACTH (as occurs in the stress response) may enhance aldosterone secretion in a minor degree. ACTH may indirectly influence aldosterone secretion by increasing the sensitivity of the adrenal gland to angiotensin II.

Tavadyan and Goncharov (1980) examined the aldosterone and cortisol levels in stressed primates. Here, they investigated the dynamics of the concentration of aldosterone and cortisol and their precursors in the blood plasma of *Macaca* rhesus. These researchers reported that the initial period of hypokinesia was characterized by a rapid and marked elevation in blood cortisol concentrations. Several days later during the hypokinesia, the amount of all steroids studied in plasma dropped below initial levels. Other investigators have also obtained similar results in laboratory animals and humans during restricted motor activity (Kolpakov, 1970; Cardus et al., 1965; Kovalenko et al., 1970). This depression of adrenal secretory activity is a manifestation of adaptation by the organism to chronic stress.

In the work of Tavadyan and Goncharov, aldosterone secretion increased rapidly to maximal levels by the second or third day of the experiment. In the latter days of the experiment, the aldosterone levels dropped to below resting levels. This result has also been observed in humans undergoing the stress of hypokinesia (Katz, 1964).

Additionally, Tavadyan and Goncharov demonstrated two phases of adrenal activity upon exposure to the stress of hypokinesia. The initial phase is described as one of stimulation or enhanced

activity of adrenal steroids followed by a second phase characterized more as an adaptation. This adaptation is a response to the
reduced demands made upon the organism.

In summary, many factors come into play to influence the secretion of aldosterone. Most applicable to the stress response is the role
the central nervous system plays in influencing the secretion of
aldosterone. Both in humans and in animals, aldosterone secretion
has been observed to generally increase as a result of the elicitation
of the stress response. Also, the increase in secretion of aldosterone
along with the increase in secretion of ADH, during stress, contributes to the water retention typically seen under conditions of
anxiety and stress.

GLUCOCORTICOIDS (Cortisol)

The primary influence of glucocorticoid activity is on intermediary metabolism. Approximately 95 percent of glucocorticoid
activity comes from the secretion of cortisol (hydrocortisone). Corticosterone and cortisone in the circulation contribute to small
amounts of glucocorticoid activity. Since cortisol exerts the greatest amount of glucocorticoid activity, the physiological effects of
cortisol, as representative of glucocorticoid activity, must be considered.

Carbohydrate Metabolism

Cortisol, an important stress hormone, exerts several physiological effects on metabolism. The most pronounced effect of cortisol
is on the liver to stimulate gluconeogenesis. Under the influence of
cortisol, the rate of gluconeogenesis can be increased to as much as
six to tenfold. The outcome of enhanced liver gluconeogenesis is a
build-up in liver glycogen storage.

Cortisol causes amino acids to be transported out from ex-
trahepatic tissues, especially from muscle. This elevates the levels of
amino acids in the blood, which results in the liver being exposed to

increasing concentrations of these organic substances. Cortisol plays an important role in enhancing amino acid transport into the liver. It also elevates the enzyme levels in the liver needed in the process of gluconeogenesis, that is, the formation of amino acids into glucose. Glucose uptake and/or metabolism is decreased in some other tissues of the body such as adipose tissue, skin, and, to some extent, muscle. As a result of the high circulating levels of cortisol, glucose concentration is elevated in the bloodstream resulting in a tendency toward hyperglycemia.

Protein Metabolism

Cortisol exerts a powerful influence on protein metabolism by causing a decrease in protein anabolism (synthesis) and an increase in protein catabolism (breakdown). This results in a decrease in the protein stores in almost all cells of the body except the liver. Liver proteins, in contrast, are markedly elevated. Loss of protein, in response to high circulating levels of cortisol, can lead to a negative nitrogen balance and ultimately to nitrogen wasting. It must be emphasized that cortisol preferentially mobilizes only labile protein constituents, rather than the basic cellular structural proteins.

Fat Metabolism

Cortisol exerts a minor influence on the mobilization of fatty acids from adipose tissue, which results in a mild increase in plasma-free fatty acid levels. Cortisol also increases cellular fatty acid oxidation. These two factors act in concert to influence metabolism in times of stress. In adipose tissue, cortisol stimulates lipolysis while promoting the lipolytic effect of epinephrine. As a result of lipolysis, the production of glycerol and lactate is also increased, which will encourage gluconeogenesis. Utilization of fats will then replace glucose as an energy source. This obviously enhances the preservation of glucose and glycogen in the body which is very much needed in times of stress.

Other Effects of Cortisol

Besides its metabolic effects, cortisol exerts profound effects on the other systems of the body.

Muscular System

It is known that the presence of glucocorticoids is necessary for maintenance of muscular strength. However, in the presence of cortisol excess, the muscular system can be weakened to such an extent that a person may not be able to stand erect.

Anti-Inflammatory Effects

Cortisol, when administered in large doses, inhibits the inflammatory response of damaged or injured tissues. It is well known that when tissues become traumatized, infected, or damaged, tissue inflammation will occur. This could be more damaging than the injury itself. Cortisol, in large enough concentrations, can inhibit this effect or even reverse the effects once inflammation has occurred. The mechanism appears to be one of stabilization of lysosome breakdown (stabilization of lysosomal membranes), and a decrease in fibroblast activity. Cortisol also decreases the permeability of the capillaries, which prevents loss of plasma into the tissues, and therefore, tissue swelling. In addition, the ability of white blood cells to reach the traumatized area and release more inflammatory substance is blocked by cortisol influence. Antibody migration and leucocycte infiltration to the traumatized area is therefore reduced.

Autoimmune System

Cortisol in large concentrations, suppresses lymphoid tissues throughout the body with a resultant decrease in lymph organ production of leucocytes, sensitized lymphocytes, and antibodies. The overall level of immunity for the organism to almost all foreign substances is diminished. Cortisol also decreases the plasma levels of eosinophils and lymphocytes. These are two types of white blood cells which play a role in providing a defense against foreign substances into the body (see Chapter 12).

The eosinophils are weak phagocytes, that is, they engulf all prevailing foreign substances. They represent approximately 1 to 3 percent of the total number of blood leucocytes. On the other hand, the lymphocytes are continuously circulating and perfusing the tissues of the body. The effect of cortisol on the white blood cell volume is immediate and lasts several hours. Indeed, an important diagnostic screening procedure to detect elevated cortisol levels is the presence of eosinopenia (small amounts of eosinophils).

In contradistinction to the effect of cortisol on white blood cells, large concentrations of cortisol enhances the production of red blood cells. The cause of this is at present unknown.

Other Tissues of the Body

Cortisol, in general, exerts an antianabolic and catabolic effect in lymphoid, bone, connective, and other tissues of the body. Cortisol may also cause an increase in the secretion of gastric juice. Further, it has been shown that cortisol is necessary for the maintenance of normal functioning of the brain. Additional effects of cortisol include its participation in the maintenance of red blood cell formation, the inhibition of DNA synthesis in some tissues, and a stimulation of the appetite.

Summary of Metabolic Effects

From the preceding discussion of the physiological effects of the glucocorticoids, it is interesting to speculate on the importance of the elevated levels of cortisol in response to stress. This phenomenon may relate to the fact that cortisol itself has profound effects on both glucose and protein metabolism. The results are markedly anabolic on liver function and either catabolic or antianabolic in other tissues. The liver is presented with the necessary metabolic substrates for the increased formation of both proteins and carbohydrates, which would place the body in excellent preparation for stressful or emergency situations. The enhanced glycogen storage in the liver may serve as a readily available reserve of energy, which can be used by the glycogenolytic hormones that are increased in the circulation in times of stress.

The added circulating amino acids, in addition to supplying the liver, may also supply any injured or traumatized tissues which may be deficient in protein because of stress.

The overall metabolic effects of glucocorticoid activity is to mobilize energy resources from tissues with an increase in glycogen storage in the liver. It goes without saying that certain tissues in the body, notably the brain, which utilizes glucose for optimal functioning, are exceptions to the glucocorticoid inhibitory effects on protein and carbohydrate metabolism.

Control of Cortisol Secretion

The zona glomerulosa of the adrenal gland appears to respond to many stimuli, which directly influence its cells to secrete hormones. Such stimuli include the blood levels of potassium, angiotensin II, and sodium. Hemorrhage is also another simuli which influences the glomerulosa to secrete its mineralocorticoids. As far as the zona fasciculata and zona reticularis of the adrenal gland are concerned, there are probably no stimuli that act directly on these cells to influence the secretion of their hormones. Adrenocorticotropic hormone secreted by the anterior pituitary gland appears to control the two inner zones of the adrenal cortex (Figure 20). A small quantity of ACTH is necessary for aldosterone secretion, although this role of ACTH is greatly overshadowed by the direct factors mentioned above.

Anterior pituitary ACTH secretion is regulated by the hypothalamic releasing hormone, corticotropin releasing hormone (CRH). Figure 20 depicts the mechanism which regulates glucocorticoid secretion. As can be seen, stressful stimuli, as registered by the hypothalamus, result in the following hormonal progression:

$$CRH \rightarrow ACTH \rightarrow Cortisol$$

This sequence of events is quite rapid. Large amounts of cortisol appear in the circulation within minutes. However, as soon as the cortisol levels in the blood become high, cortisol exerts a negative feedback on the hypothalamus to lower its CRH production and

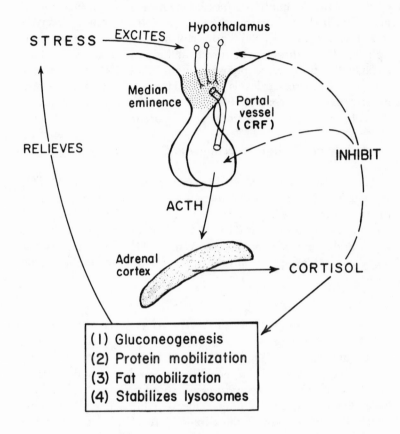

Figure 20

Illustration of the regulation of glucocorticoid secretion. Adapted from
A.C. Guyton, *Textbook of Medical Physiology*, (6th ed.). Philadelphia: W.B.
Saunders Co., 1981, p. 952.

the anterior pituitary to lower its ACTH production. Hence, a fine
control of the blood levels of cortisol and ACTH is maintained, in
order to keep these hormones at their normal levels.

The important point here is that various types of stress activate
the entire system. The outcome is the rapid and increased levels of

cortisol which promote the metabolic changes, as summarized in Figure 20. It is also important to emphasize that stimuli, perceived as a threat, can exert a very powerful influence and in their own right can break through the direct inhibiting feedback loop. This occurs when the stress is intense enough. In this case, it is conceivable to have increased levels of ACTH and cortisol without any negative feedback control. In other words, under intense stress, ACTH suppression by cortisol does not occur.

Adrenal Cortical Secretion and Circadian Rhythm

The time of day influences the secretory rates of CRH, ACTH, and cortisol. In other words, there is a 24-hour cyclic alteration in the signals from the hypothalamus that result in changes in cortisol secretion. It turns out that CRH, ACTH, and cortisol are at higher levels in the morning than in the evening. Therefore, in assessing blood cortisol levels, it is important to take into account this cyclic variation.

THE ADRENAL GLAND AND STRESS

The literature published over the past half-century has documented well the cortical and medullary responsiveness of the adrenal glands to a wide variety of stressful stimuli. Several researchers have presented overwhelming evidence which strongly demonstrates the importance of the adrenal cortex and medulla in the whole stress phenomenon. Ever since the work of Cannon (1914, 1932), Cannon and Paz (1911), and Selye (1950), special attention has been given to stress-induced adrenal responsivity by several other researchers. The extensive reviews of Mason (1968a,b,c), Mason (1972), Mason et al. (1976), Levi (1972), and Selye (1976) clearly demonstrate adrenal medullary and cortical responsivity to various types of stressful stimuli. The adrenal cortical and adrenal medullary responses to acute stress are certainly well known. Also, much research which investigates adrenal responsivity of the organism to chronic stress is described (see Selye, 1951, 1956, 1976).

Adrenal Medulla

Autonomic nervous system stimulation as a result of psychogenic-induced stimuli (arousal) is well known (Lindsley, 1951; Kopin et al., 1978). Adrenal medullary stimulation as a result of sympathetic activation induced by various psychogenic stimuli has been demonstrated by Levi (1972), Mason (1968a), Mason (1972), Roessler and Greenfield (1962), and Frankenhaeuser (1975). The physiological effects of the adrenal medullary catecholamines is described in detail by Wenger et al. (1960), and Guyton (1981).

Basically, the research of Cannon (1914, 1932) concerning the adrenal gland was described by his "fight or flight" hypothesis. The work of Cannon, as well as that of others, clearly establishes the rapid rise in circulating catecholamine levels that occurs when an organism responds to various types of stimuli. The physiological changes which accompany the elevated levels of epinephrine and norepinephrine are quite varied and subserve the "fight or flight" response.

Further, it is well known that stimuli which enhance catecholamine secretion also enhance secretion of the pituitary ACTH and adrenal corticosteroids (cortisol). However, evidence is available to suggest that under certain circumstances, the adrenal medullary response may persist longer than the adrenal cortical response, perhaps because of a more rapid adaptation by the organism to cortisol. It appears that when persistent and intense effort and alertness are required as a result of stressful stimuli the catecholamines remain elevated in the circulation in the presence or absence of cortisol.

When the catecholamines are released into the circulation, it has been observed that both epinephrine and norepinephrine are secreted together. However, recent research indicates differential secretion in these hormonal responses. Stimuli which induce increased arousal, anxiety, and apprehension in the organism are associated with increased circulatory levels of epinephrine, as compared to norepinephrine. This is similar to conditions that elevate cortisol levels in the circulation. On the other hand, increases in the secretion of norepinephrine, as compared to epinephrine, have been associated with stimuli that induce increased effort, such as physical exercise. Frankenhaeuser (1975) suggested that stressful conditions relating to general emotional arousal exhibit preferential elevations in epinephrine, while the stress of increased physical activity exhibits preferential increases in norepinephrine levels. Dimsdale and Moss (1980) subsequently demonstrated a primarily adrenal medullary response to psychological stress, while the stress of physical exercise induced a primarily sympathetic nervous system response. More specifically, these researchers demonstrated that during public speaking, epinephrine increased twofold with little change in norepinephrine, while during physical exercise, the norepinephrine levels increased threefold with a much smaller increase in epinephrine levels.

Adrenal Cortex

In all species studied, ACTH has been recognized as the primary pituitary hormone secreted as a result of various types of stress exposure (see Selye, 1950). ACTH enhances adrenal cortical activity which results in cortisol elevations in humans and corticosterone in rodents. This response to various types of stress exposures is very well documented, although some variations may occur (Mason, 1975). In addition, the hormones secreted by the adrenal cortex and their direct metabolic effects enable the organism to respond and adjust to stressful stimuli (Selye, 1950; Engel and Lebovitz, 1966).

It must be remembered that the stress response elicits the activation of several other hormonal systems besides the adrenal cortical one; all of these systems contribute toward preparing the organism physiologically to withstand and cope with stressful stimuli. The physiological preparations include not only alterations in metabolism, but cardiovascular functions as well. An example would be the influence of the adrenal medullary hormones. In the final analysis, the metabolic and other effects of the glucocorticoids discussed in this chapter may then be enhanced or counterbalanced by several other hormones which are released as a result of the elicitation of the stress response. One can sum this up by saying that cortisol, through its physiological effects, substantially increases the resistance of the body to both acute and chronic stress.

Almost any type of stress will enhance cortisol secretion by the adrenal cortex. Familiar types of stress that elevate circulating levels of cortisol include: disease states, surgery and trauma of almost any form, pain, fever, nausea, heat or cold stress, immobilization or crowding stress, invasion of the body by a foreign substance to produce infection, injection of sympathomimetic drugs into the body, hypoglycemia, apprehension, and several types of emotional conditions. However, if the adrenal cortical response to various stressful stimuli is understood from the point of view of anticipation to the stressor, significant differences in adrenal cortical secretions may be observed between different subjects. Some subjects exhibit rapid elevations in cortisol secretions, while other subjects may exhibit little, if any, response. The key here in understanding individual differences in adrenal responses to presumably identical stimuli lies in the fact that continued exposure to the same stimuli may lead to varying individual adaptive responses. As adaptation occurs, attenuation in adrenal cortical hormonal response is apt to occur. Another key issue here which may underlie the frequent variation observed in adrenal cortical response is whether the stimulus is truly perceived as stressful.

CHAPTER 7

Thyroid Gland

The thyroid gland is a two-lobed organ located just below the larynx on either side and in front of the trachea. An isthmus of thyroid tissue connects the two lobes. The adult gland weighs approximately 20 grams and is one of the most vascularized endocrine glands in the body. It has the ability to remove iodine from the blood.

Several hormones are produced by the thyroid gland which have a pronounced influence on the metabolic rates of various cells. The most important of these hormones are thyroxine (tetraiodothyronine), T_4, and tri-iodothyronine, T_3. Tri-iodothyronine is the result of removing one iodine molecule from T_4.

Assuming that all the necessary building blocks are present, the synthesis and release of these thyroid hormones are controlled by anterior pituitary thyroid-stimulating hormone (TSH) and, of course, by THRH from the hypothalamus. Thyroxine, in turn, exerts a negative feedback on TSH release.

Another hormone secreted by the thyroid gland is calcitonin (thyrocalcitonin). This hormone acts as one of the regulators of calcium levels in the blood. Due to its similarity in function to parathyroid hormone, calcitonin is discussed in the chapter describing the parathyroid gland.

PHYSIOLOGICAL EFFECTS OF THYROID HORMONES

The general effects of increased thyroid hormone concentrations in the blood include: (1) an increase in metabolism in most body cells. The exceptions include the brain, retina, lungs, spleen, and testes. Large amounts of thyroid hormone can increase the basal metabolic rate by as much as 60 to 100 percent above normal; (2) an increase in protein systhesis in almost all tissues of the body; (3) an increase in intracellular enzyme activity, and (4) an enhancement of growth of the organism mediated through an increase in protein synthesis. Excesses of thyroid hormone can, however, cause increased catabolism and mobilization of proteins rather than increased synthesis of proteins.

More specific effects of increased thyroid hormone blood levels include: (1) an acceleration of the catabolic reactions of glycolysis. Essentially, most features of carbohydrate metabolism are increased, including the rapid uptake of glucose by cells and increased gluconeogenesis (the manufacture of glucose from noncarbohydrate sources); (2) an acceleration of all features of fat metabolism. The oxidation of free fatty acids by cells with an elevation of free fatty acids in the blood is enhanced; (3) a depression of cholesterol, phospholipids, and blood triglycerides; (4) an interference with ATP synthesis in both cardiac and skeletal muscle tissue resulting in energy depletion in muscle. This occurs with excess levels of thyroid hormones; (5) an increase in the need for vitamins. This relates to the fact that vitamins form an integral part of many enzyme systems in the body. Since thyroid hormones increase enzymatic activity, the overall need for vitamins is increased; (6) an increase in body weight. This phenomenon may occur, but may be masked by an increase in appetite which may offset the change in metabolic rate; (7) an increase in oxygen utilization. This, in turn, results in an increase in the rate and depth of respiratory activity, vasodilatation in several body tissues which, in turn, increase blood flow to these tissues, an increase in the force of contraction of the heart, and an increase in heart rate with a possible slight increase in pulse pressure; (8) an increase in the secretion rate of various digestive juices and motility of the GI tract; (9) heightened activity of the central nervous system producing extreme nervousness, anxiety, and even sleeplessness, and (10) an increase in the rates of secretion of almost all of the other endocrine glands of the body.

FACTORS THAT INFLUENCE THYROID ACTIVITY

A wide variety of external stimuli or agents can alter the activity of the thyroid gland. For example, pregnancy enhances all aspects of thyroid activity due to the demands made by the fetus. Age depresses the activity of the thyroid gland, although this change may be quite small. Increased levels of the gonadal hormones may depress thyroxine transport to the tissues of the body. And finally stress, particularly that of a cold environment, stimulates thyroid hormone release.

EFFECTS OF STRESS ON THYROID FUNCTION

Various external stimuli are known to influence the activity of the thyroid gland. Any changes in TRH secretion by the hypothalamus will alter TSH secretion by the anterior pituitary. Any changes in TSH secretion will alter the output of thyroid hormones by the thyroid gland.

Cold stress is one of the well-known stimuli which significantly raises TRH and therefore TSH secretion. Thyroid hormonal output can be increased to levels well over 100 percent that of normal during cold stress. As a result, the basal metabolic rate can reach to levels as much as 50 percent above normal.

Various psychogenic stimuli also influence the secretion of TRH and TSH which in turn influence the quantity of thyroid hormone secreted by the thyroid gland. Stimuli which cause excitement and anxiety and which tend to stimulate the sympathetic nervous system seem to suppress the secretion of TSH.

Let us review some research which describes the different types of stressful stimuli on thyroid functioning.

There are several researchers who, in working with experimental animals, demonstrate that emotional or physical trauma results in increased thyroid functioning. Such authors include Bansi et al. (1953), and Eickhoff et al. (1949, 1950). On the other hand, some researchers such as Brown-Grant and Pethes (1960) demonstrate a suppression of thyroid activity. In reviewing the research protocol, several external factors must be considered which bear on the observed results. Some such factors include diurnal fluctuations, dietary regimen, and body temperature of the laboratory animals.

Other studies describing emotional stress in monkeys demonstrate stimulation of thyroid activity (Mason et al., 1961). Dohler et al. (1977), in their work, describe an activation of both the thyroid and adrenal glands after disturbance stress (laboratory maneuvers and handling of animals) in rats.

On the other hand, suppression of thyroid activity has been observed several times by exposing rats to stressful stimuli. Brown and Hedge (1973) observed a depression in TSH release accompanied by increased circulating levels of ACTH and glucocorticoids. Stressful stimuli, such as extremes in temperature, epinephrine injections, and typhoid vaccines have been shown to depress thyroid activity (Williams et al., 1949). The stress of forced exercise (Bogoroch & Timiras, 1951) and starvation (Van Middlesworth & Berry, 1951) were shown to depress thyroid activity. There are other studies in literature, dealing with experimental animals, which demonstrate a thyroid depression due to stressful stimuli. Stress-induced infection or toxemia resulting in thyroid depression have been reported by Reichlin and Glaser, 1958; Sternberg et al., 1955; and Shambaugh and Beisel, 1966.

There are several other examples that could be cited from the literature. However, to summarize the effect of acute stress on thyroid activity in the experimental animal, one may make the observation that in the majority of cases investigated, thyroid activity is suppressed. Other authors claim that no clear conclusion can be made at this time concerning the effect of emotional stress on thyroid function (Reichlin et al., 1966). For a comprehensive overview of this field, one is referred to the work of Dewhurst et al. (1968).

In considering the influence of stress on thyroid activity in humans, one finds, again, variable and conflicting results. Let us consider the stress of anesthesia and surgery in human subjects and the subsequent effects on thyroid activity. Many researchers conclude that general regional anesthesia does not affect TSH secretion in humans. Such researchers include Oyama et al. (1969), Oyama et al. (1979), Surks and Oppenheimer (1964), Goldenberg et al. (1959), Green and Goldenberg (1959), and Harland et al. (1974), among others. Most of the research in this field is concerned with the effects of anesthesia and surgery on the production, metabolism, and blood levels of the thyroid hormones. In earlier studies, indication of thyroid hormonal activity was demonstrated by measuring the protein bound iodine (PBI) levels in the blood. It must be pointed out that today, our medical technology has advanced to such a stage, that sophisticated scanning techniques are now employed to measure such changes in thyroid activity. However, it is of value here to present a brief description of the earlier research employing the measurement of PBI levels in the blood because these investigations provide us with an insight into the difficulty which such measurements entail. The complexity of such measurements, in the presence of various stressors, is reflected by the large amount of variation of responses that were observed.

Many conflicting results are seen to emerge from the literature. The early work of Perry and Gemmell (1949) demonstrates no changes in protein bound iodine (PBI) levels postoperatively after minor surgery in several patients. On the other hand, Blount and Hardy (1952) found elevations in PBI in most of their patients. These researchers also reported a decrease in PBI as well as no changes in PBI in the remaining patients in this study. Many studies dealing with the stress of surgery on thyroid activity report increases in PBI (Engstrom & Markardt, 1954; Schwartz & Roberts, 1957; and Goldenberg et al., 1955). Other researchers report no changes in levels of PBI (Charters et al., 1969; Kirby et al, 1973;

Surks & Oppenheimer, 1964), while still others report decreased levels of thyroid hormones after surgery (Burr et al., 1975).

Chan et al. (1978) also studied pituitary thyroid function during surgery. These researchers found a sharp early increase in total thyroxine level, resulting from a displacement of triiodothyronine from thyroid hormone binding proteins. The serum tri-iodothyronine levels fell rapidly during and after the operation with a concomitant rise in reverse tri-iodothyronine levels. These researchers also observed prolactin levels to increase both during and after surgery.

Ramsden et al. (1979) studied the effect of surgical stress and ACTH injection on circulating thyroxine and tri-iodothyronine levels in the rabbit. These researchers also observed prolactin levels to increase both during and after surgery. They observed that a switch from the peripheral formation of tri-iodothyronine to reverse tri-iodothyronine occurred both in normal rabbits and in rabbits with thyroxine-induced thyroid suppression. They concluded that the rabbit demonstrates changes in concentrations of serum tri-iodothyronine and reverse tri-iodothyronine after injection of ACTH or surgery similar to those seen in humans. Pollard et al. (1979) also observed a marked elevation in the tri-iodothyronine-thyroxine ratio as a result of prolonged stress in rats. These experiments certainly point to the complexity of the measurement of the stress response in terms of thyroid gland activity and necessitate the consideration of other possible intervening factors, such as catecholamine activity and glucocorticoid activation.

Several papers published by Goldenberg et al. (1954, 1955, 1956, 1957, 1959) indicate that the initial response by the thyroid gland to stress is one of stimulation. But the ensuing stress-induced increase in adrenocortical activity may be counterproductive to the peripheral effects of thyroid activity, which in turn may lead to a suppression of thyroid activity. For a much more comprehensive review of the research in this field, one is again referred to the work of Dewhurst et al. (1968).

At this point, we may review some other literature which focuses on both adrenocortical activity and thyroid functioning during stress. A study described by Ducommun et al. (1967) reports a stress-induced increase in ACTH secretion accompanied by a suppression in TSH, with a resultant decrease in thyroid activity. Yet there are other cases reported in the literature in which this response was not observed (D'Angelo, 1960a, b; and Sakiz & Guillemin, 1965).

In the work of Langer and Lichardus (1969), thyroid activity and its fluctuations during and after several acute stresses such as trauma, dehydration, adrenalectomy, is viewed in the light of dexamethasone administration in rats. These researchers found a decrease in thyroid function after an initial inhibitory period. These authors contend that the observed increase in thyroid activity as a delayed response to stress may partly elucidate the mechanism involved in the increased thyroid function consequent upon emotional stress and other stresses, as is sometimes seen in humans and animals.

In terms of other acute stressful stimuli in humans such as athletics, disturbing interviews, fear-provoking films, and sensory deprivation, a situation of thyroid stimulation is generally observed with no significant alterations in thyroid function. In all these cases, individual differences as well as the degree of intensity of the stressor are some of the external factors which add to the variation and complexity of the results.

SUMMARY

There are numerous studies to date concerned with the stress-induced changes in pituitary thyroid function. From a very brief overview of the above-mentioned research, it is clear that more investigative work is necessary in order to elucidate the complex relationships which exist between various categories and degrees of stressful stimuli and thyroid function. External variables which closely relate to thyroid function and thyroid hormone metabolism must be considered as an integral part of any investigative work in this area. Such variables include individual differences, sex, age, and nutritional status. Also, the roles of sympathetic stimulation, adrenal medullary secretion, levels of circulating catecholamines and glucocorticoids released as a result of the stress response, along with their concomitant stimulation or inhibition of thyroid gland activity, should be considered.

It may be stated at this point that in the experimental animal a brief but transient elevation in thyroid activity is sometimes observed as a result of acute stress. Whether this is a result of alterations in TSH secretion is not known at present. However, from much of the available research, it can be concluded that subsequent to the onset of emotional and physical stresses in animals, a rapid suppression in thyroid activity is observed. This observation correlates well with the rapid decrease in the secretion of TSH.

It was also observed from the above brief literature review that thyroid activity may increase following certain stresses both in animals and in humans. This is definitely so in the case of cold stress.

In order to substantiate the results for other types of stresses, at least in the human, it must first be understood that the studies in which these results are based are very difficult to control. Again the extreme ranges in individual differences, individual reactivities, and precise measurement of human thyroid function must not only form an integral part of these studies, but must be very precisely controlled. This is necessary in order more accurately to assess the observed results of stress.

CHAPTER 8

Parathyroid Gland

PARATHYROID HORMONE

Located on the posterior surface of the thyroid gland are the glands of the parathyroid, usually four, two associated with each of the lateral lobes of the thyroid. The glands secrete a hormone known as parathormone, or parathyroid hormone (PTH). This hormone regulates the calcium and phosphate levels in the bloodstream by exerting an influence on the transport properties of these ions on the tissues of bone, kidney, and intestine. PTH exerts its effect on the intestine by enhancing the absorption of calcium and phosphate. PTH also acts directly on bone by causing an increase in the number of osteoclasts, causing the removal of inorganic substance from bone, which results in a rise in the blood levels of blood calcium and phosphate. PTH acts on the kidney by increasing the reabsorption of calcium and increasing the excretion of phosphate. This occurs in direct proportion to the levels of PTH in the bloodstream. The effect of PTH in influencing these three organ systems, plus the effects on calcium and phosphate as a result of intake, metabolism, and excretion, all contribute to maintaining the plasma levels of calcium and phosphate within normal limits.

The secretion of PTH is not regulated by the hypothalamus. Instead, release of PTH occurs by means of a negative feedback loop between the blood calcium levels and the parathyroid glands. As blood levels of calcium rise, PTH secretion is depressed. On the other hand, parathyroid hormone secretion is increased when blood calcium levels are depressed.

CALCITONIN

As mentioned previously, calcitonin (thyrocalcitonin) is a hormone secreted by the thyroid gland which also functions to regulate the calcium levels in the blood. This hormone acts to lower blood calcium levels by regulating the rate at which calcium leaves bone tissue and enters the extracellular fluid compartment. Calcitonin acts in reverse to parathormone.

Calcitonin secretion is thought to be directly controlled by the blood levels of calcium. As calcium blood levels decrease, calcitonin secretion is decreased. As calcium blood levels increase, calcitonin secretion is increased, thereby lowering blood calcium concentration.

CALCIUM AND STRESS

There is very little evidence to date to indicate that stress may directly influence the secretion of parathyroid hormone or calcitonin. However, stress may exert an indirect effect on these hormones by influencing the calcium levels in the blood. There is research available, although sparse, to indicate that various types of stress may influence circulating calcium levels, both in laboratory animals and in humans. Let us now briefly review some research in this field.

Calcium under conditions of stress has been studied by some researchers from both an intracellular and extracellular vantage point. Intracellular calcium has been studied by Cheah and Cheah (1976) in terms of mitochondrial calcium efflux. These researchers first reported varying rates of mitochondrial calcium (Ca^{++}) efflux in different breeds of pigs. In their work they suggest that Ca^{++} efflux may be linked to stress-susceptibility. In a subsequent work, they correlated rates of mitochondrial Ca^{++} efflux with parameters closely related with porcine stress susceptibility (Cheah & Cheah, 1979). These researchers worked with two stress syndromes found in certain kinds of pigs. The stress-related conditions they studied include malignant hyperthermia and a condition associated with muscle wasting in which rapid glycolysis post-mortem occurs. Malignant hyperthermia results in muscular rigidity, tachycardia, hyperventilation, and severe metabolic acidosis. These researchers found a significant increase in mitochondrial Ca^{++} efflux during malignant hyperthermia induced by halothane. Also, with regard to the condition of muscle wasting, the rates of Ca^{++} efflux and glycolysis were shown to be in direct proportion. Muscles exhibiting rapid glycolysis were associated with high Ca^{++} mitochondrial efflux rates, while low Ca^{++} efflux rates were associated with muscles having a slow glycolysis rate. These observations were made only on post-mortem samples. From their work, these authors concluded that the rates of mitochondrial Ca^{++} efflux correlated highly with parameters associated with procine stress, in conditions of malignant hyperthermia and of rapid glycolysis in muscle. The mitochondrial Ca^{++} efflux rates were also directly related to the rate of hydrolysis of creatine phosphate and of adenosine triphosphate (ATP) (Cheah & Cheah, 1979). It is well known that ATP and creatine phosphate are of paramount importance in acting as a coupling agent for energy transfer in cells. Both substances contain high energy phosphate bonds. However, creatine phosphate is several times more abundant in muscle. These same authors (Cheah & Cheah, 1976) postulated that the calcium released from the mitochondria of stress susceptible pigs may be the responsible agent inducing post-mortem rapid glycolysis. Ca^{++} has the ability to activate myofibrillar ATPase and phosphorylase kinase causing more glycogen to be converted into lactate (glycolysis).

The condition of restraint stress on serum calcium and phosphate was studied by a number of other researchers. In preliminary studies, it was found that in both intact (Schwille et al., 1974) and thyroidectomized rats (Schwille et al., 1975), hypocalcemia occurred. Hofmann et al. (1979) also investigated restraint stress both in normal and thyroidectomized rats. These researchers found that in the intact and thyroidectomized rats, serum total calcium, ionized calcium, and previously injected radioactive calcium, decreased after 8 hours of severe restraint stress. The stress restraint model they used consisted of periods of weak electric shocks (Schwille et al., 1977). The results of the study of Hofmann et al. (1979) showed that there is a distinct stress-induced decrease of both total calcium and ionized calcium levels in rats left intact, and in rats which have been thyroidectomized. In both intact and thyroidectomized rats, when compared to control, the stress-induced decreases in calcium were shown to be significant. Also, for both intact rats and thyroidectomized rats, these researchers observed significant increases in inorganic phosphate in stress-induced rats as compared to control rats. Essentially, their results demonstrated that rats after restraint-induced stress are associated with hypocalcemia and hyperphosphatemia.

Tigranian et al. (1980) studied extracellular calcium levels in humans undergoing stressful conditions. These researchers worked with male students before and immediately after an examination, and studied the levels of parathyroid hormone (PTH) and calcium. They found the pre-examination blood levels of PTH and calcium to be either increased or at the upper normal limit. After the examination, they found no significant changes in PTH but calcium levels were significantly increased.

SUMMARY

Stress-induced malignant hyperthermia and rapid glycolysis in muscle increased mitochondrial Ca^{++} efflux in laboratory animals. Also, some researchers found hypocalcemia to occur after restraint stress in both intact and thyroidectomized animals. On the other hand, calcium levels were found to be increased after psychogenic-induced stress in humans. However, general findings seem to point to a stress-induced decrease in calcium levels in the blood. Any observed increases in calcium levels as a result of stress remain unexplained, but perhaps may be attributed to the possible rapid loss of calcium from cells.

It might be added here that there are other factors which may influence calcium absorption. These factors may or may not play a role in the altered physiology associated with the elicitation of the stress response.

Growth hormone can increase calcium absorption, thereby increasing the levels of calcium in the blood. It is known that in many instances the secretion of GH is increased as a result of the stress response. Perhaps the higher circulating levels of GH may influence calcium levels in the blood by increasing its absorption and producing a hypercalcemic effect. At this point, this is highly speculative. Other hormones may influence the levels of calcium in the blood. For example, the thyroid hormone, thyroxine, plays an important role in bone formation, and may exert an influence on the calcium levels in the blood. Also, thyroxine in high doses may inhibit or increase the secretion of calcium into the gut. The glucocorticoids may exert a similar effect on calcium levels in the blood.

An obvious factor that may also influence calcium levels is the daily dietary intake. Certainly, a diet previously low in calcium may stimulate an increase in its absorption.

The interrelationships between these calcium controlling factors as well as others (low intestinal pH, lactose in the diet) and the implication for the stress response yet remain to be clarified.

CHAPTER 9

Reproductive Glands

The reproductive functions in both the male and female are substantially controlled by the hormones of the anterior pituitary gland and the sex glands, namely the testes in the male and the ovaries in the female.

Anterior pituitary gonadotropin (FSH, LH) secretion, while quiescent during the early years of childhood, begins to change around the ages of ten to twelve, leading to increased secretions of these hormones. The mechanisms that initiate such changes in the developing male and female are not well known. What is known, however, is that the gonadotropin-releasing hormone (GnRH or LHRH) from the hypothalamus is released, and this in turn influences anterior pituitary release of two glycoprotein hormones, namely, follicle-stimulating hormone (FSH) and luteinizing hormone (LH), into the general circulation. These hormones reach their target tissues, the sex glands, in order to exert their specific physiological effects.

MALE HORMONES

In the male, FSH is responsible for the onset of spermatogenesis. LH stimulates the testes to produce the most important male hormone, testosterone. For this reason, LH is also called interstitial cell stimulating hormone (ICSH), since it stimulates the activities of the interstitial cells. These cells are responsible for the production of testosterone.

Testosterone is the most important male hormone produced. Androgens which are produced by the adrenal gland are also male hormones, but taken together, their potency does not approach that of testosterone. Testosterone is responsible for the development and maintenance of the male secondary sex characteristics. Testosterone is also needed during the final stages of spermatogenesis where it exerts its influence.

Testosterone production acts to regulate the secretion of the pituitary gonadotropins. The effect is one of inhibition, and it is a negative feedback control system that operates continuously, to exert a very fine control over testosterone levels in the blood. In essence, testosterone in the blood feeds back to the hypothalamus, thus inhibiting the release of LHRH. This mechanism sets a limit upon the rate at which testosterone is produced.

EFFECTS OF STRESS ON MALE SEX HORMONES

The overall effect of stress on plasma testosterone levels is one of suppression. This has been observed both in animals and humans (Selye, 1976). The exact mechanisms which elicit such a response are as yet to be clarified. It is suggested that stress may interfere either at a central or peripheral level. The central action of stress would of course occur at the hypothalamic-hypophyseal levels. Peripherally, stress may act directly at the level of the gonads or on testosterone metabolism itself. Most of the data available, which investigate the phenomenon of stress-induced testosterone suppression, indicate the direction to be predominantly a central mediated action of stress. In some unknown way, stress affects the hypothalamic-pituitary gonadal axis, or perhaps even some extrahypo-thalamic pathways.

In their work, Taché et al. (1980) found that adult male rats, after immobilization stress applied for 6 hours daily for a duration of 6 days, increased their plasma corticosterone levels, and decreased testosterone and prolactin levels significantly. The gonadotropin, luteinizing hormone (LH) was also mildly suppressed. These same workers studied the condition of adrenalectomy and found that basal levels of testosterone, prolactin, and LH, were not modified in any way. However, in adrenalectomized animals under the same situation of immobilization stress, testosterone and LH levels were both suppressed, whereas the concentration of prolactin was elevated, particularly when compared to nonadrenalectomized animals. Taché et al. (1980) concluded that the increase in glucocorticoid secretions during chronic restraint exposure may play a role in the prolactin decrease but not in the decrease of LH and testosterone. Also, through binding studies using (^{125}I) Iodo-HCG (human chorionic gonadotropin), they concluded that the suppression of testosterone after immobilization stress is not mediated at the level of the testes. It is well known that there are specific membrane receptors in the Ledig cells of the rat, which bind HCG or LH. Both these hormones in turn stimulate testosterone secretion (Catt et al., 1976). Taché et al. (1980) found that after immobilization stress, rats showed no modification in HCG binding capacity or in the testosterone response to HCG. Since the suppression of testosterone after immobilization stress is not mediated at the level of the gonads, it may involve a more central mediated response, namely the hypothalamic-pituitary level. Since it is known that LH plays a role in the regulation of testosterone secretion, the LH suppression, which also occurs after immobilization stress, may be partially related to testosterone suppression. Also, Saez et al. (1977) showed that the number of HCG binding sites and the steroidogenic function of the testes is suppressed under the influence of the in-vivo administration of glucocorticoids. It also appears that the testosterone decrease is related more to the LH decrease and not to any role played by the gonadotropin, follicle stimulating hormone (FSH), and prolactin. Taché et al. (1976, 1978, 1979) and Du Ruisseau et al. (1977, 1978) have also shown that under various other conditions of stress-induced increase of glucocorticoids, there is a concomitant suppression of LH, FSH, and prolactin secretions.

To summarize, the work of Taché et al. (1980) suggests that testosterone suppression following immobilization stress seems to be mediated chiefly at a central level. Also, the sustained presence of glucocorticoids due to immobilization stress may not play an important role in LH and testosterone levels but may influence prolactin suppression. Further, testosterone suppression may be linked more to LH suppressed levels rather than to FSH and prolactin levels. FSH and prolactin levels do not seem to play important roles with regard to testosterone levels.

In addition, according to Taché et al. (1980), while testosterone levels remain significantly depressed, LH levels gradually tend to return toward basal levels after 6 days of stress. Also Ellis et al. (1976), Nakashima et al. (1975), and Aono et al. (1976), in their work dealing with chronic stress, reported that while testosterone levels remain low, LH may not change significantly, or may even rise. All of these observations indicate that while LH may play an important role in stress-induced testosterone suppression, the possibility that other factors may be involved should not be ruled out.

On the other hand, Tigranian et al. (1980) studied a situation involving 15 male students, aged twenty-eight to fifty-five years, under conditions of emotional stress. Emotional stress was induced by the taking of a state examination of internal medicine in medical school. Blood samples were taken before the examination and immediately after successful passing. The subjects were uninformed in advance about the study, and their agreement was obtained immediately after the first blood sample was taken. It was found that before the examination, the levels of FSH, LH, and testosterone were normal, but after the examination, all three hormones showed a significant elevation. The authors explain that the increase in the levels of LH, FSH, and testosterone, which occurred after the examination, may result from a general anabolic effect of these hormones, particularly in response to the demands made on the body during emotional stress. Several other researchers have also found plasma testosterone levels to be suppressed after chronic psychogenic or somatic stress. This has been shown for both animals and human subjects. For example, in humans, testosterone suppression was found to occur in situations involving major surgical interventions, intensive exercise, or fear-evoking situations (Kreuz et al., 1972; Aono et al., 1976; Carstensen et al., 1973; Ellis et al., 1976; and Davidson et al., 1978). Also, immobilization, surgery, and crowding have been reported to decrease plasma testosterone levels in animals (Gray et al., 1978; Rose et al., 1972; Repcekova & Milulaj, 1977; Bliss et al., 1972; and Bardin & Peterson, 1967).

Other researchers have also found LH levels to be suppressed concomitant with testosterone levels. The work of Gray et al. (1978) demonstrated that chronic surgical stress in rats resulted in a suppression of testosterone levels, accompanied in most cases by a decrease in LH levels. Ellis et al. (1976) found a decrease in LH and testosterone levels in patients undergoing surgery. Carstensen et al. (1973) demonstrated a decrease in LH and testosterone in patients undergoing surgery, and in particular, they observed that plasma LH and testosterone levels decreased 4 to 5 hours after surgery. However, over a continuous 24-hour interval, testosterone levels remained suppressed while LH levels returned to normal.

Other researchers who have found a significant depression in the plasma levels of testosterone during and immediately following surgery include Charters et al. (1969); Matsumoto et al. (1970); Monden et al. (1972); and Tanaka et al. (1970).

A study of the relationship between testosterone and ACTH secretion was pioneered by Sorcini et al. (1963) and Conti et al. (1963). These researchers demonstrated that ACTH administration in males significantly reduced the levels of testosterone in the plasma. In a later work, Sorcini et al. (1974) demonstrated that an increase in ACTH levels during surgery coincided with a decrease in plasma testosterone levels. Along with the increase in ACTH, they reported that there was also a concomitant increase in the levels of plasma LH. These authors concluded that the increase in ACTH is responsible for testosterone depression both during and after surgery. Still other researchers demonstrated that the indirect effects of ACTH stimulation on adrenal androgen and progesterone production could influence the suppression of LH secretion (Andrews, 1970; Christian, 1971; Lisk, 1969; and Thomas & Gerall, 1969).

Another study concerned with the effects of acute stress on the secretion of LH, FSH, growth hormone, and prolactin in the normal male rat, warrants mention. Krulich et al. (1974) subjected male rats to a variety of stresses such as simple handling of the animals, transfer of animals from room to room, ether anesthesia either alone or combined with bleeding of the animals, the injection of saline or epinephrine, and the condition of restraint. Subsequent to each of the stressful stimuli, LH, FSH, growth hormone, and prolactin secretions were investigated. It was found that all of these hormones varied in terms of their sensitivity of response to the stressful stimuli mentioned above. These researchers observed a distinct elevation in prolactin secretion and a decrease in GH secretion. The response of LH varied. LH exhibited an initial elevation in secretion which was frequently followed by a decrease in its secretion. FSH seemed to remain least affected. Therefore, in terms of sensitivity to response, these researchers found prolactin and growth hormone secretions to be most sensitive, the secretion of LH to be less sensitive, and FSH, the least sensitive.

Another study concerns itself with the influence of maternal stress on the development of the male fetal genital system. Dahlöf et al. (1978) exposed rat mothers to various types of stress stimuli during the last trimester of pregnancy. The types of stress exposure involved in this study included crowding, cold, and immobilization-illumination stress. It was found that at birth the male offspring had a decreased anogenital separation. Also, these researchers observed that the mothers exposed to the stress of immobilization-illumination or cold stress, produced offspring with reduced body weight and reduced weight of the testes and adrenal glands. These authors state that the corticosteroid secretions of the stressed mother may play a role in the gonadal depressed secretions of the male fetus.

Summary

In general, it has been found that following exposure to stressful stimuli, testosterone levels are depressed. From the research work cited, it has been demonstrated that the stress associated with surgery, immobilization, and crowding result in a depression of plasma testosterone in animals. In work with humans, it has been shown that the stress of major surgical procedures, intensive exercise, combat training, and the emotion of fear result in lowered plasma testosterone levels. The above-mentioned research has also pointed to the fact that the decreased plasma testosterone levels during stress occur in the presence of normal circulating levels in LH. Testosterone suppression during stress does not appear to be mediated by suppressed levels of LH or FSH. The role of ACTH in influencing suppression of testosterone has also been reviewed.

FEMALE HORMONES

The hormonal hierarchial system in the female resembles that of the male with the exception of two major hormones, namely, estrogen and progesterone. These hormones are secreted by the ovaries in response to anterior pituitary and hypothalamic gonadotropin activity. The various hormones are secreted in different amounts at different times during the monthly female sexual cycle. It is believed that all the female hormones including LH, FSH, and LHRH undergo cyclic variation.

The gonadotropin hormones, LH and FSH, perform a similar function in the female as they do in the male. In the female, they function in the monthly development of the ovarian follicles. LH, in particular, is responsible for final follicular growth and ovulation.

The estrogens and progesterones form the two basic groups of female sex hormones. Several female sex hormones are secreted not only by the ovaries, but by other tissues such as the adrenal cortex, and the placenta (during pregnancy). However, in the nonpregnant female, the primary source of estrogen is the ovaries. Like testosterone in the male, estrogen is primarily responsible for the development and maintenance of female secondary characteristics and for the growth of specific body cells.

Progesterone, on the other hand, performs its primary role during the preparation of the uterus for pregnancy and in preparing the mammary glands for the process of lactation.

The female sex hormones constantly feed back to the hypothalamus to inhibit or excite LHRH secretion. The inhibition or excitation of LHRH is a function of the cycle phase. During the postovulatory part of the cycle (the time between ovulation and the onset of menstruation), estrogen and progesterone production together inhibit hypothalamic LHRH release. This results in a strong negative feedback depression of both FSH and LH release by the anterior pituitary. Before menstruation occurs, involution of the corpus luteum takes place and estrogen and progesterone secretion fall to low values. The decreased levels of these hormones release the previous negative feedback inhibition on the hypothalamus, and this results in an increase in secretion of both LH and FSH. Both gonadotropins are at elevated levels in the circulation. The presence of the high circulating levels of the gonadotropins enhances the development of new ovarian follicles. As the follicles grow, they continue to secrete estrogen until its concentration increases to more than six times its previous low levels. During the first 12 days of follicle development, and under the high levels of estrogen secretion, LH and FSH slowly decrease in secretion. Approximately 12 days after the initiation of menstruation, the secretory pattern of fall in LH and FSH suddenly reverses itself and a preovulatory surge in both LH and FSH occurs. Estrogen is at a high level at this time and appears suddenly to exert a positive feedback effect on the hypothalamus. This may explain the overwhelming surge in LH and, to a lesser extent, the surge in FSH secretion that now occurs. This surge in LH leads to ovulation and corpus luteum formation. A new cyclic round of the female hormonal secretions then ensues (Guyton, 1981).

The gonadotropins are also sensitive to various nervous stimuli which reach the hypothalamus from other sources. There are many types of nervous stimuli which exist that influence the secretion of the gonadotropins. For example, in sheep and goats, nervous stimuli which result from climatic variations, or the amount of daylight, influence gonadotropin secretion on a seasonal basis. Psychic stimuli can also influence gonadotropin secretion in animals. This is true in the human as well, where various psychogenically induced stimuli are known to cause pronounced excitation or inhibition of gonadotropin secretion. For example, the female monthly cycle is greatly affected by various psychological stimuli and environmental factors. Stress can be seen to play an important role in influencing female hormonal production through alteration of gonadotropin secretion.

EFFECTS OF STRESS ON FEMALE SEX HORMONES

Let us review some research concerning the effect of stressful stimuli on female hormonal secretions. There is documented research concerning the effects of stressful stimuli on the ovarian cycle in the human female. The effects of psychogenic stress are reported in a work described by Peyser et al. (1973). These researchers observed that stressful stimuli strongly influence the menstrual cycle. Subjects were hospitalized after three normal menstrual cycles so that the preovulatory surge in LH could be assessed under controlled conditions. Increased levels of hydroxycorticoids were found in each subject upon hospitalization, and these levels were found to decrease when the subjects were allowed to go home. The midcycle preovulatory surge in LH and ovulation was found to be delayed in these subjects.

Abplanalp et al. (1977) studied cortisol and growth hormone responsivity to psychological stress during one menstrual cycle in 21 healthy subjects in order to see if these hormones were related to estrogen levels. The results of their study demonstrated that the cortisol and GH responses to psychogenic stress were a function of anxiety levels in these subjects, but were not a function of the menstrual cycle phase. Therefore, cortisol and GH levels were not related to the varying estrogen levels during the cycle.

On the other hand, a study describing subjects who were using or not using oral contraceptives, and who were exposed to the psychogenic stress of self-evaluation during varying stages of the menstrual cycle, was investigated by Marinari et al. (1976). These researchers observed that adrenocortical responsivity to psychogenically induced stress was significantly greater in subjects tested during the premenstrual phase of the menstrual cycle than in those subjects who were tested during the midcycle phase of the menstrual cycle. Also, no such differences in adrenocortical responsivity as a function of the phase of the cycle was observed in subjects who were using oral contraceptives. These authors speculate that responsivity to psychological stress may be a function of the magnitude of fluctuations of the gonadotropin hormones during the menstrual cycle. The greater adrenocortical responsivity seen in this study during the premenstrual phase points to the presence of a heightened and marked physiological reactivity to stress. Thus, the work of Marinari et al. (1976) suggests that a premenstrual increase in physiological reactivity to psychogenic stress is present in subjects experiencing a normal menstrual cycle, as compared to those subjects using oral contraceptives. This result should be considered in view of the fact that several researchers have found cortisol levels to be relatively stable throughout the course of the menstrual cycle (Aubert et al., 1971; Saxena et al., 1974; and Genazzani et al., 1975). With regard to animal research, it might be added that Nequin and Schwartz (1971) studied the stress of barbitol anesthesia administration in female rats and its effect on ovulation. They observed a significant delay in ovulation in rats subjected to this condition.

An interesting perspective is to review the interrelationships which exist between the effects of psychogenic stress, estrogens, and the cardiovascular system. Several researchers (von Eiff & Piekarski, 1977; and von Eiff et al., 1971) have reported that during psychogenically induced stress, the estrogens in the female play a role in lowering the cardiovascular response to blood pressure and heart rate. De Loos et al. (1979) performed experiments in the rat which were focused on investigating the role of the sex steroids on heart rate, in response to acute emotional stress. These researchers found clear indications that the secretion of ovarian hormones, during the oestrous cycle, depresses the heart rate reaction to emotional stress. They concluded that the presence of the female sex hormones, whether estrogen and/or progesterone, in physiological quantities, plays an important role in the reaction of the cardiovascular system to emotional stress.

Along the same line, there is also evidence to suggest that sex hormones may perform important functions in the regulation of peripheral blood flow and the organism's reactivity to overall systemic vascular stress. At present, there is evidence to indicate that the presence of estrogens may account for the low occurrence of atherosclerotic lesions found in the female as compared to the male. Interestingly enough, the incidence of atherosclerotic lesions is about equal in males and females of similar ages, provided the females have reached menopause. It is well known that menopause is characterized as a state of depressed circulating levels of estrogens.

PROLACTIN

This hormone is secreted by the anterior pituitary gland and promotes the secretion of milk by the mammary glands. It is the hypothalamus which functions to control prolactin secretion, but this control differs from its control over the other anterior pituitary hormones, in that it mainly inhibits prolactin release. As mentioned previously, both hypothalamic releasing hormones, PRH and PIH, regulate prolactin secretion, yet it is PIH that plays the more dominant role. PIH may itself be the familiar catecholamine, dopamine, which is known to be secreted in the hypothalamus, and which also can decrease the production of pituitary prolactin secretion.

Prolactin is a hormone which is secreted by the pituitary gland of the pregnant mother, and its circulating levels rise steadily from the fifth week of pregnancy until the birth of the baby. At this time, it increases to extremely high levels in the circulation, often as high as 10 times the normal level. After the birth of the baby, prolactin plays an important role in the process of lactation. It enhances milk secretion. The hormone prolactin is also present in the male in smaller quantities, but its predominant function in the male is not known.

It has been observed that stress has a pronounced effect on prolactin secretion.

EFFECTS OF STRESS ON PROLACTIN SECRETION

It is well known that prolactin secretion is enhanced by many types of stressful stimuli (Euker et al., 1975; Krulich et al., 1974; Frantz et al., 1972; Turpen et al., 1976; and Noel et al., 1972). Such stimuli include ether anesthesia (Ajika et al., 1972; Krulich et al., 1974; Riegle et al., 1976; Turpen et al., 1976; Valverde-R. et al., 1973; Piercy & Shin, 1980; and Shin, 1979), cold stress (Jobin et al., 1975), immobilization stress (Krulich et al., 1974; Riegle et al., 1976; and Taché et al., 1978) and surgical stress (Neill et al., 1970; and Riegle et al., 1976).

It seems that almost any type of physical or emotional stress results in a surge of prolactin secretion (Frantz et al., 1972). Also, prolactin levels are elevated in the blood even when patients are examined by doctors (Koninckx, 1978).

It is thought that the enhanced secretion of prolactin during stress is a result of the stimulation of PRH, or inhibition of PIH, or a combination of both reactions. In fact, Shin (1979) presents evidence that the prolactin surge which occurs during ether stress seems to be a result of the stimulation of PRH rather than of inhibition of PIH.

Blizard et al. (1977) investigated those factors which correlate basal serum prolactin levels with individual susceptibility to stress. These researchers present further evidence that prolactin may indeed play a funcional role in the response by the organism to stressful stimuli.

Other hormones have been shown to influence prolactin secretion. Estrogen is stimulatory to prolactin release (Piercy & Shin,

1980; Ajika et al., 1972; Chen & Meites, 1970; Kalra et al., 1973; Ratner et al., 1963; and Shin, 1979).

Thyrotropin releasing hormone (TRH) has been shown to stimulate prolactin secretion in the female and in estrogen primed rats (Piercy & Shin, 1980; and Stevens & Lawson, 1977) but not significantly in male rats (Piercy et al., 1980; Lu et al., 1972; Shin, 1978; and Stevens & Lawson, 1977). Information on the relationship between TRH and prolactin secretion during stress is sparse. However, a study relating the stress associated with parachute jumping and the secretions of prolactin, TRH, and GH is described by Noel et al. (1976). These researchers found that prolactin, TSH, and GH are released in physiologically significant amounts following the initial stressful condition of parachute jumping. The significance of these hormonal elevations for normal physiological functioning remains to be elucidated in full.

The role of the endogenous opioids in mediating prolactin release is another interesting area of present investigative work. The enhancement of prolactin secretion, as influenced by morphine, was first suggested by Meites et al. (1963). Subsequently, Tolis et al. (1975) and Rivier et al. (1977), along with several other researchers, demonstrated the morphine-induced stimulation of prolactin release in both humans and animals. The endogenous opioids in question include the enkephalins and β-endorphins. Naloxone is a drug known to be a specific opiate antagonist. It has been demonstrated by several researchers that noloxone is effective in inhibiting a rise in prolactin secretion (Rivier et al., 1977; Meltzer et al., 1978; and Brown et al., 1978). Stress-induced prolactin elevation in rats has been shown by several researchers, including Ferland et al. (1978), Rossier et al. (1980), and Van Vugt (1978). Other studies show no such effect (Rivier et al., 1977 and Martin et al., 1979). Ragavan and Frantz (1981) present a study describing the suppression of serum prolactin by naloxone but not by anti-β-endorphin antiserum in stressed and unstressed rats. They concluded from their studies that the endogenous opioids are to some extent involved in both the tonic and stress-induced increase in prolactin secretion, and serve as one of many mechanisms involved in the regulation of prolactin release.

SUMMARY

As reviewed in the text, the secretion of all the gonadal hormones fall into a very fine delicate sequence of interrelationships. A subtle balance exists between the hypothalamic releasing hormones, the anterior pituitary gonadotropins, and the ovarian sex hormones. For example, in terms of the events which lead to the onset of ovulation, one first observes the hypothalamic secretion of LHRH followed by the release of the anterior pituitary gonadotropins. Subsequent to this, the ovarian female sex hormones are secreted, which in turn is followed by ovulation. Throughout the cycle, this delicate balance of hormonal interrelationships persists. The role of the hormone prolactin in the cycle is not known. However, inputs from the central nervous system, such as information pertaining to external stimuli, can interfere with this fine balance. It is well known that almost any type of intense stress can interfere with the menstrual cycle, sometimes to the point of amenorrhea. During emotional distress, the monthly cycle in many women will be altered or even stopped for a short period of time. For example, emotional reactivity to such conditions as embarking on a journey, a life crisis situation such as a separation or death of a loved one, a divorce or even the onset of various types of psychiatric disturbances such as acute depression, commonly result in amenorrhea.

One can then appreciate the difficulty involved in assessing all these hormonal levels along with their interrelationships. To add to the difficulty, the hormones are subject to continuing diurnal fluctuations. To study the alteration in this hormonal balance as a result of the elicitation of the stress response is indeed an arduous task.

The female hormonal levels of estrogens, progesterone, and the gonadotropins have been observed to be influenced in one manner or another by stressful stimuli. Also, there is now much documented research to indicate that stressful stimuli do exert an effect on prolactin secretion. Some stressful stimuli that induce elevations in prolactin release have been discussed. Specific examples include the rise seen in prolactin secretion during surgical procedures. For example, procedures such as gastroscopy and even a gynecologic examination are associated with increased levels of prolactin. However, during physical exercise and after venipuncture, prolactin levels do not seem to be affected. Some studies relating the effects of psychogenic stimuli on elevations in prolactin secretion are also available. Motion sickness is seen to elevate plasma prolactin levels. Also, the physiological cyclic elevations in plasma prolactin that accompanies nursing is a well-known observation.

It must be stated that the physiological and behavioral role in the surge of prolactin, as well as the variations in the other female hormones as a result of stress, is not well understood. More specifically, the mechanisms involved in the phenomenon of stress-induced prolactin secretion remain to be elucidated.

CHAPTER 10

Pancreas

The pancreas is located along the greater curvature of the stomach. It empties its contents through a single duct called the pancreatic duct, right into the small intestine with the common bile duct. In this respect, the pancreas functions as an exocrine gland, in that it secretes its digestive juices through a duct. However, it also functions as an endocrine gland because it releases its hormones directly into the blood stream. The endocrine portion of the gland is made up of cell groups called the islets of Langerhans. Two distinct cell types are present in the islets, the alpha and beta cells. The alpha cells secrete the hormone glucagon and the beta cells secrete the hormone insulin.

GLUCAGON

Glucagon is a protein hormone which stimulates the conversion of stored glycogen in the liver and muscle to glucose (glycogenolysis). This causes the level of glucose in the blood to be elevated.

Hence, glucagon is sometimes referred to as a hyperglycemic agent. It is well known that the catecholamine, epinephrine, also elevates blood glucose levels; however, the activity of glucagon in raising blood sugar is much more effective than epinephrine.

GLUCAGON AND STRESS

In general, the elicitation of the stress response results in an elevation of glucagon secretion. In particular, stressful conditions which result in hypoglycemia stimulate the secretion of glucagon. A case in point is fasting. Most researchers agree that glucagon levels are elevated in human plasma during fasting conditions. There may be a slight blunting effect on glucagon elevations in this condition due in part to the release of free fatty acids into the bloodstream. It has been observed that free fatty acid levels are elevated during fasting, and they appear to inhibit glucagon secretion. However, the cumulative effect appears to be one of glucagon elevation.

It may be stated that stress, in general, results in an elevated secretion of glucagon from the pancreas. Such an elevation enhances glycogen breakdown, and gluconeogenesis. These processes both contribute toward keeping sugar levels high, which provide nourishment and energy for the organism during the time of stress.

INSULIN

Insulin is a protein hormone whose major activity is to lower blood glucose levels. It has the exact opposite effect on glucose as does glucagon. In essence, this hormone is known to produce two major effects: (1) It increases the uptake of glucose by certain cells of the body. Some of the tissues affected by insulin include cardiac, skeletal and smooth muscle, liver, and adipose tissue; and (2) It stimulates the conversion of glucose into glycogen (glycogenesis), particularly by liver and muscle cells. Other effects of insulin include the promoting of amino acid transport into cells and the enhancement of protein and fat synthesis.

Both glucagon and insulin secretion are regulated by a negative feedback mechanism. Blood sugar levels influence the secretion rates of both hormones. When glucose blood level falls, glucagon is secreted and insulin secretion is depressed. When glucose blood level rises, insulin is secreted and glucagon secretion is depressed. Both hormones function together to maintain a relatively constant blood sugar level despite great variability in carbohydrate intake.

INSULIN AND STRESS

The most direct determinant of insulin secretion is the glucose levels in the blood. For example, a rise in blood sugar level above a critical level of about 80 to 100 mg/100 ml. stimulates a rapid secretion of insulin. The subsequent decrease in sugar levels inhibits the further release of insulin. However, the negative feedback relationship between blood glucose levels and insulin is modulated by several other hormones and even metabolites. Let us consider those factors that are stimulatory to insulin secretion, either directly on insulin itself, or indirectly on insulin, through a primary influence on blood glucose levels.

Growth hormone can both directly stimulate insulin secretion and indirectly stimulate insulin secretion, by primarily raising blood sugar levels. Growth hormone is known to raise blood sugar levels by affecting liver enzymes and enhancing the release of glucose from the liver. It is known that GH is increased during the stress response. GH is one of many hormones that elevates blood sugar and perhaps any extra insulin that may be secreted as a result of the increased blood sugar levels is necessary to keep blood sugar levels in check.

Thyroxine, like growth hormone, raises blood sugar by affecting liver enzymes and enhancing release of glucose from the liver. Hence it has an indirect affect on the secretion of insulin.

Cortisol also enhances glucose release from the liver. Cortisol enhances blood sugar levels by inhibiting peripheral insulin-induced glucose uptake. Cortisol may also directly influence insulin secretion, but the response time is slow.

In an emergency situation, that is, during stress, epinephrine stimulates a quick increase in glucose levels in the blood. It may mediate this effect by: (1) decreasing insulin-stimulated glucose uptake by muscle; and (2) an α-adrenergic effect, that is, a direct inhibition of pancreatic insulin secretion. It appears that the β-cells of the pancreas are adrenergically innervated.

All of these hormones, that is, growth hormone, thyroxine, cortisol, glucagon, and epinephrine, promote hyperglycemia and are the hormones that are increased in secretion during the stress response. Since they elevate blood sugar, they therefore tend to stimulate the secretion of insulin. Epinephrine, on the other hand, through α-adrenergic activity, inhibits insulin secretion. Since these hormones are secreted during the stress response, one may ask, what is the net effect of these hormonal interactions on insulin secretion? The net effect of all these hormones is a function of the state of the organism, particularly in terms of its already existing levels of blood glucose. For example, if the state of the organism is one of hypoglycemia, blood sugar levels may rise without any elevations in insulin secretion, provided the blood sugar levels do not rise above a critical level. Likewise depending on conditions, insulin secretion may be lowered when blood glucose levels are lowered.

There are other factors which play a role in stimulating insulin secretion.

The rise of amino acids in the circulation generally increases insulin secretion relatively independently of elevated blood glucose levels.

Elevated levels of free fatty acids in the blood influence insulin secretion by depression of insulin-induced glucose transport into muscle. The outcome is elevated glucose levels and enhanced insulin secrtion.

Also, nervous stimuli of various sorts may influence insulin secretion. The role that the nervous system plays in infuencing insulin secretion remains to be clarified.

Let us now consider some situations which are inhibitory to insulin secretion. It is well known that insulin secretion is depressed under conditions of low blood glucose. The two well known physiological states in which this occurs are exercise and fasting. These states present a situation of stress to the organism. Also, any α-adrenergic agent acts to inhibit insulin secretion. The important catecholamine and adrenal medullary hormone, epinephrine, which is elevated in the blood during the stress response, acts to inhibit insulin secretion. Perhaps some of the decreased levels of insulin observed in these states of fasting and exercise may result from the presence of epinephrine rather than from lowered blood glucose levels.

Also, another hormone that exerts an inhibitory influence on insulin is angiotensin II. It is well known that angiotensin II is a potent vasoconstrictor agent and may well be elevated during the elicitation of the stress response. The integrating mechanisms involved here are not too clear.

Another curious finding relates to the fact that diurnal fluctuations have been observed in circulating levels of insulin, seemingly unrelated to blood glucose levels.

Figure 21 summarizes the various factors that influence insulin secretion. The several factors listed show either an excitatory or inhibitory effect on insulin secretion. In general, the effect of acute stress is one of depression of insulin secretion.

Let us review some recent literature describing the alterations in insulin and glucagon secretion under various stressful conditions.

Brockman and Manns (1976) investigated a condition of acute trauma such as liver biopsy, in which portal plasma glucagon and insulin concentrations were measured in conscious sheep. These researchers found that this condition enhanced glucagon secretion while depressing insulin secretion. Due to this altered hormonal status, they found, as expected, the presence of hyperglycemia.

It is known that insulin inhibits glucose production and enhances the rate of glucose removal from the blood (West & Passey, 1967). Also it is known that glucagon is a potent glycogenolytic agent and potent gluconeogenic agent in humans. This hormone has also been shown to be a potent glycogenolytic agent and to enhance hepatic gluconeogenesis in sheep (Brockman & Bergman, 1975). This activity of glucagon may account in part for the elevated blood sugar levels observed by Brockman and Manns (1976) in their studies. Also, the researchers found that in spite of the presence of

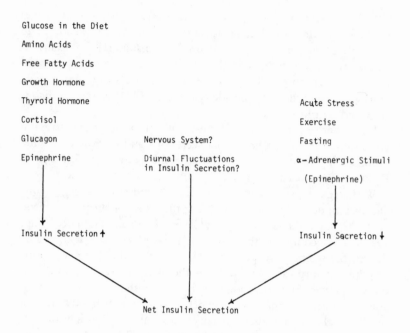

Figure 21

Factors that influence net insulin secretion.

hyperglycemia, the insulin concentrations remained depressed. The depressed insulin concentrations must also contribute to the observed hyperglycemia. This was the case also in another group of animals which received additional glucagon infusion. These same researchers found that not only was the trauma of liver biopsy sufficient to depress plasma insulin concentrations, but also the infusion of glucagon was not sufficient to prevent the stress inhibition of insulin secretion.

Brockman and Manns (1976) also concluded from their studies that the hormonal changes which produce the hyperglycemic state may also involve, in part, the sympathetic nervous system. This is also confirmed by other researchers, such as Phillips et al. (1969). These researchers concluded that the catecholamines are required for the pancreas to promote hyperglycemia.

Other researchers such as Yamaguchi and Matsuoka (1982) studied the effect of electric stress (electrical shocks) in rats, and found that a decrease of glucose-stimulated insulin release occurred. These researchers concluded that this insulin depression produced by a combination of a high fat diet and electric stress may in part involve the inhibition of the adenylcyclase cAMP system, which is activated by glucose.

Still other researchers have found that trauma and other stressful conditions may affect hormonal secretions and carbohydrate metabolism in the anesthetized animal (Ashby et al., 1965; Nijjar & Perry, 1971; and Bloom et al., 1973).

With regard to humans, it has been found that hyperglycemia and insulin depression occurs during the stress of surgery (Allison et al., 1969; Giddings et al., 1977; Clarke, 1970; and Halter & Pflug, 1980). To account for the observed hyperglycemia which occurs during the stress of surgery, it is known that the neuroendocrine response to surgical stress involves the increased secretion of various hormones. Such hormones include growth hormone, cortisol, and the catecholamines, all of which may play a distinctive role in the hyperglycemia response (Ichikawa et al., 1971; Newsome & Rose, 1971; Noel et al., 1972; Halter et al., 1977; and Madsen et al., 1978). However, Halter et al. (1977), in an effort to explain insulin depression, state that this depression may stem from two possible causes, one related to the anesthesia type used, and one related to the neuroendocrine adrenal medullary response, possibly induced by afferent pain signals from the site of the traumatized tissue.

SUMMARY

When viewed from a broad perspective, the secretion of insulin is controlled by several factors. The most relevant factors include those that are related to carbohydrate metabolism and those that are not. When viewed from the point of view of the stress response, insulin secretion is influenced by such factors as relate to blood glucose levels and the levels of other stress hormones.

As indicated, the level of glucose in the circulating bloodstream appears to be quite a strong controlling factor in regulating the secretion of insulin. Hence, whatever substances that directly affect glucose levels in the blood will also exert an influence on insulin secretion.

The hormones, epinephrine, growth hormone, thyroxine, cortisol, and glucagon, generally appear to increase in the circulation as a result of the elicitation of the stress response. All of these hormones have the effect of elevating the level of glucose in the blood. Hence all of these hormones are stimulatory to insulin secretion due to their influence in elevating the level of blood glucose. In addition, the hormones, glucagon and growth hormone can exert a direct stimulatory effect on insulin secretion while epinephrine can exert a direct inhibitory influence on insulin secretion. Angiotensin II is another hormone which may exert an inhibitory influence on insulin secretion. Its effect as well as the effect of a diurnal variation of insulin levels in the blood, independent of glucose levels, remains to be elucidated. Also, the presence of metabolites such as elevated levels of amino acids and free fatty acids in the circulation enhance the secretion of insulin. Gastrointestinal hormones, such as gastrin, pancreozymin and secretin have also been shown to enhance insulin secretion when injected. There is some evidence to indicate that both hormones, pancreozymin and secretin, may stimulate insulin secretion under physiological conditions. There are other factors such as sympathetic nervous system activation and other stimuli originating in the nervous system which may influence the secretion of insulin. On the other hand, exercise, fasting, the hormone epinephrine, and any condition of acute stress, generally all act to depress insulin secretion.

The net effect of all these factors on insulin secretion, both under normal conditions and as a result of the elicitation of the stress response, depend, in the final analysis, on the physiological state of the organism.

In view of the above, it is obvious, that the secretion of insulin is controlled by a multiple of factors, most of which are related to the circulating levels of glucose in the blood, which in turn, is related to the amount of glucose intake and to carbohydrate metabolism.

CHAPTER 11

The Pineal Gland

The pineal gland, also termed the epiphysis, is located deep between the cerebral hemispheres on the posterior aspect of the mid-brain. Some cells of the pineal appear to receive innervation from postganglionic nerve fibers of the sympathetic nervous system. Impulse conduction on these fibers appears to stimulate certain pineal cellular activity.

Several chemically and physiologically active substances have been isolated from the pineal gland. These substances include the hormones, melatonin, norepinephrine, and serotonin. The chemical substance, histamine, has also been isolated from the pineal gland. Melatonin is the only substance that is actually synthesized by the pineal gland. Melatonin secretion appears to be a function of the amount of light received by the eye. As the amount of light detected changes, the secretion of melatonin changes in proportion.

Melatonin has the ability to cause the clustering of pigment granules of the skin, particularly in lower animals. As earlier noted, this phenomenon results in a darkening of the skin surface and may serve as a camouflage mechanism to act as a protective device for animals against adverse environments.

Melatonin is also thought to play an important role in the regulation of reproduction and sexual function in lower animals. It influences the release of certain hypothalamic releasing hormones which, in turn, regulate the secretion of adrenocorticotropin hormone (ACTH) and the gonadotropins, FSH and LH, by the anterior pituitary. The role of the pineal gland in melatonin secretion, reproduction, and sexual function in humans, remains to be clarified.

EFFECTS OF STRESS ON THE PINEAL GLAND

Let us review some research concerned with the pineal gland under the influence of stress. Kvetnansky et al. (1979) studied the effects of immobilization stress on the levels of epinephrine, norepinephrine, and dopamine in the pineal gland in the rat. These researchers found an increase in the epinephrine content of the pineal gland in the stressed animal as compared to control animals. Increases in norepinephrine and dopamine were not found. These researchers noted that since epinephrine is the major catecholamine released by the adrenal medulla into the circulation in increased amounts during stress, it may be possible for epinephrine to be taken up by the pineal gland. It has been found that in stressed animals, the pineal nerves contain much more epinephrine than norepinephrine, the opposite of what is normally the case.

There is some evidence to indicate that the uptake of epinephrine may occur in the pineal sympathetic nerves. Previous work has shown that the pineal can take up and retain more epinephrine than the other tissues or organs innervated by the sympathetic nervous system (Steinman et al., 1969). If indeed the pineal nerves contain more epinephrine than norepinephrine in the stressed animal, then sympathetic stimulation will result in both epinephrine and norepinephrine release. Hence, under conditions of stress, β-receptor stimulation, which is more sensitive to epinephrine than to norepinephrine, will be enhanced while α-receptor stimulation may be diminished. Hence, the physiological effects on end-organ activity will be altered since the α- and β-receptors are known to have, in certain cases, different or opposing effects (refer to Table

II). These same researchers have also observed a similar epineph-
rine-norepinephrine exchange in the sympathetic nerves of the
heart. The increase in epinephrine content of rat hearts was again
observed during immobilization stress.

As for stress-induced melatonin secretion by the rat pineal,
Lynch et al. (1973a, 1977) and Vaughan et al. (1978a) demonstrated
an increase in the synthesis of this pineal hormone. However,
Vaughan et al. (1979), during various short-term conditions of
stress, found no change in melatonin secretion in humans. These
researchers concluded that the normal stresses of day-to-day living
probably do not exert any major effects on the pineal secretion of
melatonin.

On the other hand, Wetterberg (1978) and Lynch et al. (1978)
investigated the effect of prolonged exposure on shifted cycles of
light-dark and wakefulness-sleep and found alterations in the
rhythmical secretions of human melatonin.

The pineal gland has also been studied from the point of view of
chronic auditory stress exposure and ulcer disease in humans. For a
review of the pineal gland in relation to the neuroendocrine aspects
of chronic auditory stress and ulcer disease, including ultrastruc-
tural studies of the pineal gland, the reader is referred to the work
reported by Miline (1980).

Also, evidence is available which demonstrates the influence of
pineal function on neoplastic disease (Lapin, 1976). Treatment with
pineal melatonin has been shown to be inhibitory for growth of
some cancer cells (Buswell, 1975) but not of others (Huxley and
Tapp, 1972; Bostelmann et al., 1971). Other researchers have
shown that pineal extract administration can inhibit tumor growth
to some degree (Huxley & Tapp, 1972; Bindoni et al., 1976; and De
Marzo et al., 1958). Quay and Gorray (1980) also investigated
pineal influence on tumor growth. These authors presented evidence which demonstrates that pineal influence on tumor growth
may be mediated by the effects of the pineal gland on metabolism
and glucose homeostasis. Evidence is also presented which indicates that pineal influence on tumor growth, mediated by hormonal
secretions and alterations in metabolism, may be a function of certain circadian rhythms of the host organism.

CIRCADIAN RHYTHM

The pineal gland is also thought to regulate certain patterns, fluctuations, or rhythms of specific hormonal secretions and other chemical substances. This is familiarly known as circadian rhythm. Examples of circadian rhythm include: (1) the pineal may influence the anterior pituitary ACTH secretions, which fluctuate according to the time of day; (2) the pineal may function in the regulation of the female reproductive cycle by exerting a cyclic influence on the secretions of the hypothalamic gonadotropin releasing hormones; and (3) the pineal may influence the familiar patterns of repeated behavior which is associated with diurnal cycles, i.e., the cycles of day and night, and also patterns of behavior associated with seasonal changes. For example, during the winter months, the pineal gland secretions are inhibitory to the secretion of gonadotropins from the anterior pituitary in lower animals. The gonads then become dysfunctional. But during the months of spring, the pineal inhibitory effect on the gonadotropins is lost, and the gonads become functional again.

EFFECTS OF STRESS ON CIRCADIAN RHYTHM

Circadian rhythms of various hormones and other chemical substances are characterized by a 24-hour cycle, and is a subject of investigation by many researchers.

The circadian rhythm of the pituitary-adrenal system is probably the most well established of cyclic neuroendocrine activities. Humans, as well as most animals, demonstrate rhythms in the secretion of the pituitary adrenal system over a 24-hour period, with the highest levels occuring prior to awakening, and the lowest levels occuring toward the end of the day (Krieger, 1975).

Disruptions in circadian rhythms have been shown on occasion to produce unpleasant side-effects, such as sleepiness and fatigue. Traveling long distances has been shown to alter natural circadian rhythms (Sollberger, 1965) possibly mediated through the light and dark cycle. Also, it is generally thought that the circadian rhythms influence the blood levels of certain endogenous compounds and their urinary excretion patterns (Sollberger, 1965; and Halberg, 1969). It is known that circadian rhythms exist for various clinically relevant parameters (Kanabrocki et al., 1974; Halberg et al., 1959, among others).

One of the major parameters influencing circadian rhythms is stress (Selye, 1950). Steinbach et al. (1976) demonstrated that the rhythmic patterns of such parameters as blood glucose, blood leukocytes, and body temperature, are markedly influenced by stress. Brodan et al. (1982) investigated the effects of four different types of stressors on circadian rhythms. These researchers studied the effects of sleep deprivation, fasting, isolation, and cardiac catheterization in humans. They found marked changes in circadian rhythms as a result of the presence of stressful conditions. Moreover, the alterations in the circadian rhythms increased with the duration of the stress. These researchers claim that changes in circadian rhythms may serve as a tool in assessing both the presence and intensity of a stressor.

Factors influencing the pituitary-adrenal rhythms and their variations in terms of stress responsiveness has been studied by Taylor et al. (1976). These researchers studied the highest and lowest secretion levels of the pituitary-adrenal rhythmical cycles, and modified these rhythms by the application of various types of stressors. They observed a diminished stress responsiveness at the peak of the cycle. Available evidence for the source of regulation of the hypophyseal-adrenal circadian rhythms points to the central nervous system (Krieger, 1974; and Dunn, 1974).

SUMMARY

The phenomenon of circadian rhythm was reviewed. It was noted that certain rhythmical patterns can indeed be disrupted by various types of stress exposure.

As far as the pineal gland is concerned, the phenomenon of stress may also include not only the role of the hypothalamic-hypophyseal-adrenal axis but also the epithalamo-epiphysial (pineal) axis.

Regarding the stress response, it appears that the pineal gland is distinct in function to the pituitary gland, almost acting in an opposing manner to the increased activity of the hypothalamic-hypophyseal axis. The pineal gland seems to be more sensitive to sensory stimuli from the environment such as light, dark, and noise. In its hormonal response to these sensory stimuli, the pineal gland may act asa modulating factor to the activity of the hypothalamic-hypophy-seal-adrenal system during stress. In summary, the neuroendocrine regulatory mechanisms of the pineal gland are aimed to protect the organism against disturbing and hostile environments. Its protective influence may indeed play an important role in the balance and endurance of the organism during various types of stress exposures.

CHAPTER 12

The Immune System

Endocrinology and immunology are two closely related physiological systems. Throughout all the organs and tissues of the body, they interrelate in manifold ways. While most of the previous discussions have been devoted to the alterations that take place in the endocrinological systems of the body as a result of the elicitation of the stress response, we find that it is the alterations in the immunological system that occur as a result of stress, that in recent years, have been slowly gaining widespread attention. Therefore, the following discussion is devoted to a general description of the basic physiology associated with the immune system, followed by a review of some recent literature describing the effects of various types of stress exposure on the immunological responsivity of the body.

The defense of the body to foreign invaders can occur by means of various mechanisms, some nonspecific, and some specific. Enzyme activity, inflammation, interferon, and phagocytosis are some of the nonspecific methods employed by the body to create a defensive barrier against foreign substances. More specific methods include the development of a certain type of resistance known as immunity. Here, the body builds up a defense system to combat specific foreign intruders such as pathogens, or the toxins they may release. Among the elements that appear to play an important role in the immunity of the body include certain types of blood cells, the lymphatic system, the spleen, and the thymus gland.

WHITE BLOOD CELLS

There are six different types of white blood cells (leukocytes) which are normally found in the blood. These include neutrophils, eosinophils, basophils, monocytes, lymphocytes and plasma cells. The blood also contains great numbers of cells called platelets, which can be viewed as fragments of a seventh type of white blood cell. Since the platelets do not function in a direct role as far as the immune system is concerned, they will not be discussed here. Let us briefly describe some of the above-mentioned white blood cell types that are commonly found in the circulation.

The neutrophils and the monocytes possess the mobility to pass in between the cells of blood vessel walls. This enables them to travel from the bloodstream into any tissue which an invading foreign substance might have penetrated. The neutrophils have the ability to "eat" or engulf (phagocytize) small particles. The monocytes are able to do this with larger particles.

The eosinophils comprise only a few percent of the total number of blood leucocytes. They are at most weak phagocytes. They seem to be present in the body along the tissues of the lungs and digestive tract where several foreign proteins generally pass through the body. The eosinophils are thought to attack or detoxify these proteins before they cause any harm to the body. The eosinophils are also thought to help in phagocytizing the end-products of antigen-antibody reactions. The eosinophils also seem to be related to some specific immunological adaptive reactions, particularly allergy. It has been observed that when a person suffers from asthma, hay fever, or other allergens, the number of eosinophils markedly increases. As a result of the elicitation of the stress response, it is known that the number of eosinophils greatly decreases.

The basophils travel in the circulating blood and cause the release of heparin. Heparin is a substance which can depress and even prevent the blood from coagulating. Histamine, serotonin, and bradykinen, are other substances that the basophils, along with the mast cells, can release into inflamed tissue areas.

The lymphocytes attack foreign proteins (antigens) and are briefly discussed below in the section describing the lymphatic system.

LYMPHATIC SYSTEM

The lymphatic system consists of several vessels which transport fluids (lymph) from the interstitial spaces which surround the cells of the body into the blood vessels. It appears that the lymphatic system works in conjunction with the circulatory system, to assist in the circulation of body fluids. The various vessels of the lymphatic system generally lead to specialized structures called lymph nodes. The lymphatic vessels not only transport fluids which surround various tissue cells, but also transport many foreign substances such as microorganisms and toxins which may somehow have found their way into tissue fluids. These fluids, as mentioned previously, are transported to the various lymph nodes located along lymphatic vessels throughout the body. The lymph nodes, also known as lymph glands, contain large amounts of lymphocytes which play an important role in the immunological mechanisms of the body. The lymph nodes, as well as other tissues of the body, produce lymphocytes which specifically protect the body against foreign agents such as bacteria and viruses. The lymph nodes also contain various types of phagocytic cells which engulf foreign matter, as well as the remnants of old and worn out cells.

Large amounts of other immunologically competent lymphocytes are produced by the bone marrow and the thymus gland.

Lymphocytes with antigen responsivity capabilities are also produced through the mediation of humoral antibodies. However, at present there is no known organ in mammals that functions specifically to produce these antibodies.

SPLEEN

The spleen is situated in the upper left portion of the abdominal cavity and is located behind the stomach and below the diaphragm. It can be considered the largest lymphatic organ in the body. There are several blood vessels which supply the spleen and feed into the various venous sinuses that comprise this organ. The spleen can serve as a huge blood bank, and its reservoir of blood is filled or emptied depending on the needs and activities demanded by the body. For example, during periods of stress, such as exercise or hemorrhage, the blood vessels constrict and some of the stored blood is emptied into the circulation. During stress, it is as if the spleen, in anticipation of blood loss, contracts and adds volume as well as numbers of red blood cells into the blood stream. Simultaneously, the coagulability of the blood also increases.

Part of the spleen is also composed of lymphatic tissue similar to that found in the lymph nodes. In this tissue, one finds large numbers of lymphocytes and phagocytes. Again, the lymphocytes help to defend the body against foreign invaders, and the phagocytes, as in the case of the spleen, engulf worn out red blood cells, and other cellular debris. The spleen then performs a function similar to that of the lymph nodes, that is, it acts to filter blood in the same way the lymph nodes filter lymph.

THYMUS GLAND

The thymus gland is a two-lobed organ located in the mediastinum behind the sternum, in front of the aorta, and between the lungs. This gland is larger in children as compared to adults. During growth of the organism, the size of the thymus appears to diminish. In an elderly person, it may be small and is often largely replaced by connective tissue.

There is very little doubt that the thymus gland secretes substances that are true hormones. These hormones, just as in the case of the other endocrine glands, are secreted into the blood stream, circulate throughout the body, and reach remote target tissues, where they exert their physiological effects. The thymus is thought to secrete a hormone called thymosin which plays a role in influencing the production of certain white blood cells called lymphocytes. Another hormone of the thymus gland is thymopoietin. It is a polypeptide hormone which is secreted by the epithelial cells of the thymus. It is thought to play a role in the differentiation of precursor type lymphoid cells. Still another hormone, called promine, is also thought to be secreted by the thymus, and it plays a role in promoting cellular reproduction and growth.

The thymus gland itself is comprised of lymphatic tissue subdivided into lobules. These lobules contain large amounts of lymphocytes, and together with lymphocytes from other parts of the lymphatic system in the body, play an important role in the immunity of the organism against the invasion of foreign substances. In essence, the thymus gland is seen to function as an endocrine gland, while at the same time it exerts a prominent role in the immunological mechanisms of the body. Its role in immunological functioning can be viewed in terms of the development of a "strain" of lymphocytes. For example, the thymus gland receives some lymphocytes which have been released from the bone marrow. These lymphocytes are still in the undifferentiated state when they reach the thymus. Within the thymus gland, the undifferentiated lymphocytes experience various stages of development and alterations and become T-lymphocytes. The name T-lymphocytes is to be distinguished from those lymphocytes called B-lymphocytes, which are derived from the bone marrow and which never migrate to the thymus gland. Both lymphocyte types travel throughout the bloodstream and finally take up residence in various lymphatic tissues of the body.

THE IMMUNE SYSTEM AND STRESS

There are several studies which demonstrate that emotional stress can exert an influence on the immunological mechanisms of the body (Rasmussen, 1969; Amkraut et al., 1971; Solomon, 1969; and Johnson et al., 1963).

Amkraut et al. (1971) observed in animals that were emotionally stressed an increase in the development of autoimmune diseases. Solomon (1969) demonstrated a depression of antibody synthesis in animals who were emotionally stressed. Other studies demonstrate a depression of homograft rejection (Rasmussen, 1969) and an increase in the susceptibility to infection (Johnson et al., 1963) in animals that were emotionally stressed. However, the mechanisms underlying these responses remain to be clarified. With regard to the etiology of certain disease states, such as infectious disease, autoimmune disease, and allergy, alterations in the immunological mechanisms have been clearly implicated. The degree of emotional stress, in modifying the pathogenesis of such disease states, is a subject of intense inquiry (Solomon & Moos, 1964).

Other researchers have demonstrated that hormonal responses may clearly interact with the immune mechanism. For example, Hadden et al. (1970), MacManus et al. (1971), and Nowell (1962) have demonstrated that the catecholamine, epinephrine, can exert an influence on lymphocyte metabolism in vitro.

Joasoo and McKenzie (1976) studied the effects of emotional stress, as a result of overcrowding or isolation, and the administration of exogenous epinephrine in immunized animals. These researchers measured the in vitro responses of the rat spleen lymphocytes to antigen. They observed a depressed lymphocyte response to antigen in animals that were injected with epinephrine, and in male rats undergoing the stress of either isolation or crowding, as compared to control animals. However, in their study, female rats exhibited an increase in an in vitro response of sensitized spleen lymphocytes to antigen during crowding, and a decrease in response during isolation. In this study, a sex differentiation in immune response was noted. Other researchers had also previously demonstrated a sex variation in immune response (Tobach & Bloch, 1956).

Bonnyns and McKenzie (1979) studied rat peripheral lymphocyte responsiveness to plant mitogens and found that stress in intact rats clearly influenced lymphocyte responsiveness to the plant pathogen.

Several studies have been performed which relate hormonal interactions and immunoreactivity. For example, it is known that various hormonal systems have a regulatory role with respect to lymphoid tissue. Adrenocorticotropin hormone is known to depress production of antibodies (Elliot & Sinclair, 1968). Other researchers have observed growth hormone to play a positive role in immunological development and expression (Pierpaoli et al., 1970; and Fabris et al., 1970). Gisler and Schenkel-Hulliger (1971) studied the influence of hormonal regulation on the immune response under stressful conditions in the laboratory animal. These researchers exposed mice to acceleration stress, ether anesthesia, or ACTH injection. They found that the reaction to antigen in vivo was poor at the time that spleen cells were explanted during high circulating levels of the corticosteroids. Immune responsivity was depressed by corticosterone, but the immune responsivity was increased in the presence of growth hormone.

On the other hand, Monjan and Collector (1977) demonstrated that the effect of environmental stressors on laboratory mice can not only depress immune responsivity, but also increase it. These researchers demonstrated that the levels of cortisol in the plasma appeared to be related to the depressed immune response, but not the elevated response. The mechanism involved in this latter phenomenon is open for further study.

Studies have also been performed which demonstrate a relationship between tumor growth and stress. Sklar et al. (1981) studied the growth of a transplanted mastocytoma following acute and chronic physical stress in mice. As found in earlier studies (Sklar & Anisman, 1979; 1980), a single acute shock, 1 day after tumor cell transplantation, promoted its growth. Application of the same stressor, 5 or 10 days after cell transplantation, also accelerated tumor growth. However, these researchers found that controllable shock given on each of 1, 5, or 10 consecutive days after cell transplantation had no effect on tumor growth. The implication is that the influence on tumor growth is a function of the ability to cope with stress. The tumorigenic effects of stress appear to be subject to the process of stress adaptation. There are also several other studies which report the depressive effects on tumor growth after exposure to chronic stress (Burchfield et al., 1978; Newberry et al., 1976; Rashkis, 1952; and Zimel et al., 1977).

Pavlidis and Chirigos (1980) also studied the stress-induced impairment of macrophage tumoricidal function. These researchers exposed mice to acute immobilization stress. They found that macrophages from mice, exposed to stress, showed a decreased immunoresponsiveness. They further observed that the corticosteroids were able to exert an inhibitory influence on macrophage cytotoxity. On the other hand, Riley (1975) reported a study in which mice with mammary tumors were exposed to different degrees of chronic stress. The results of the study suggest that intermittent or moderate chronic stress appears to predispose these mice to an increased risk of mammary carcinoma. This response may be mediated through a compromise in the underlying immunological mechanism responsible for host resistance and protection to hostile environments.

Sklar and Anisman (1980) studied the growth of syngeneic mastocytoma in male mice, following exposure to both physical and social stress. These researchers reported that social isolation, following tumor cell transplantation, exacerbated tumor growth. They also reported that the abrupt changes in social conditions, rather than the isolation itself, appeared to be at the root of enhanced tumorigenicity. Another finding demonstrated that the behavior patterns of the animals, after social change, could modify tumor growth. However, in mice who were engaged in persistent fighting, the tumorigenic effects of social change were not apparent. In all of these studies, Sklar and Anisman (1980) suggest that various factors must be considered, in order to comprehend the inconsistent effects of stress exposure on tumorigenicity that have been reported in the literature. Such factors include the degree of coping responsivity, stress chronicity, as well as the social conditions of the animals, both prior to and during stress exposure. For a description of further investigative work relating tumorigenicity, immunoresponsivity, and stress exposure, the reader is referred to Riley (1981).

A study by Udupa et al. (1980) considers the role of stress in the development and progress of carcinoma in various parts of the body. These researchers discuss the possible roles of the corticosteroids and catecholamines, secreted during psychogenic-induced stress, on carcinoma development. The immunosuppression caused by cortisol could lead to the proliferation of mutant cells, which in turn may lead to tumor growth. These researchers postulate that the catecholamines, through their vasoconstrictive effects, particularly on a (genetically) weak organ, may lead to an anerobic environment, with subsequent transformation of normal cells into abnormal cells. Under immunosuppression, the abnormal cells could develop into cancerous growths. Wick (1977, 1978) has also implicated catecholamine interference on the influence of tumor development.

Decreased responsivity to mitogens or antigens have also been reported to occur in humans as a result of stress exposure (Eskola et al., 1978).

SUMMARY

It is now a well-known fact that, as a result of the elicitation of the stress response, the hypothalamic-hypopyseal-adrenocortical axis is stimulated. Increased amounts of ACTH, released by the anterior pituitary, enhance the release of glucocorticoids (cortisol) by the adrenal cortex. Cortisol in large amounts profoundly influences the various blood cell types found in the circulation. For example, under high circulating levels of cortisol, depression of neutrophil motility occurs. The eosinophil count is depressed (eosinopenia). The number of lymphocytes is also decreased (lymphocytopenia). This is due to an increase in maturation and a decrease in differentiation of the lymphocytes themselves. Further, the tissues which contain lymphocytes shrink or involute. Examples include the shrinking or the contraction (loss of tissue mass) of the spleen and the involution of the thymus gland, observed as a result of stress, extended into its chronic phase. The lymph nodes, in particular the peripheral lymph nodes, and other lymphatic structures throughout the body, have also been observed to decrease in size, as a result of stress. This has been described as stress-induced atrophy of the thymicolymphatic organs.

In reviewing the literature concerned with the effects of various types of stress and the immunological response, it should be kept in mind that while much of the work was done on the laboratory animal, these models certainly should be viewed as having some application to humans. Also, the difficulties involved in establishing control conditions could be at the basis of many conflicting reports in some earlier studies.

Also, in reviewing the outcome of several research studies, some of which may demonstrate contradictory results, one should consider the conditions of stress exposure, the types of stress, the ability to control stress, as well as the chronicity of stress, as important parameters which contribute to the variability in individual responsivity.

The reports cited above, as well as several others that are found in the literature, clearly present evidence that stress, probably mediated through endocrinological alterations, can exert an interference effect on the immune response, which results in alterations in immunological functioning. As described, studies are available which report adrenal cortical influence on immunosuppression as well as catecholaminergic influence on tumor development.

Also, tumor growth or rejection does not necessarily reflect the operation of immune functioning or the immune system in the body. This is so, because tumor growth can be directly influenced by physiological factors such as blood flow, the presence of steroids, and other hormones which are generally increased in the circulation as a result of stress. It should be noted therefore that there are well known mechanisms in which stress can directly influence tumor growth without affecting the immune system.

The many studies reported in the literature point to an increased emphasis in examining the interrelationships which exist between stress and the immune mechanisms. This leads to the further development of a new scientific discipline, namely psychoneuroimmunology (Ader, 1981). This may very well parallel the more familiar study of the interrelationships that exist between psychogenically induced stress and its influence on hormonal regulation, namely psychoneuroendocrinology. Perhaps in time both these disciplines will be developed to a point where they may be viewed from a more integrative and unifying perspective.

CHAPTER 13

Other Hormonal Systems

RENIN-ANGIOTENSIN SYSTEM

The most powerful vasoconstrictor agent in the body is angiotensin II, and the precursor to its production is renin. The kidneys are stimulated to secrete the hormone renin, when the level of sodium in the extracellular fluids of the body is depressed, or when there is a drop in intravascular volume, and the blood flow to the kidneys is decreased.

When renin is secreted, it acts on a plasma substrate (plasma protein) to form angiotensin I. A converting enzyme then acts to convert angiotensin I to a potent vasoactive agent known as angiotensin II. This hormone plays an important role in the control and regulation of arterial blood pressure. Its presence causes the renal arterioles to constrict. This results in renal retention of both salt and water, increasing extracellular fluid volume, which in turn elevates arterial pressure. Angiotensin II, or simply angiotensin, also causes pronounced peripheral arteriolar constriction and moderate constriction of the veins. This phenomenon can lead to a decrease in the intravascular volume.

Angiotensin, besides being a potent vasoconstrictor agent, also plays a role in stimulating the adrenal cortex to release aldosterone. It may be recalled that aldosterone is a hormone that regulates the sodium concentrations in the body fluids. Both renin and angiotensin may exert a direct influence on the kidneys, in order to enhance sodium and water reabsorption. These hormones may promote fluid reabsorption by acting directly on the kidney tubules (similar to the action of antidiuretic hormone), or by influencing renal blood flow through their vasoconstrictive activities.

In addition, there are several humoral agents that may act to modulate renin activity. Such agents include ACTH, ADH, the adrenal catecholamines, steroid hormones, and the main electrolytes of plasma. ACTH acts to enhance the sensitivity of the adrenal gland to angiotensin, thereby exerting a small indirect effect on aldosterone secretion.

Renin secretion may occur not only as a result of a decrease in blood volume, as cited above, but also from sympathetic nervous system activity, mediated by the central nervous system on aldosterone secretion. It is known that the stress of pain and anxiety, acting through neural mechanism, enhances aldosterone secretion. The β-adrenergic stimuli and enhanced sympathetic nervous system activity also increase renin secretion. The factors that play a role in stimulating renin, angiotensin, and aldosterone, are summarized in Figure 22.

Renin-Angiotensin System and Stress

The influence of the sympathetic nervous system and the pituitary adrenocortical system on renin secretion certainly implicates this hormone in the stress response. Various stressors have been shown to elevate the circulating levels of renin in animals undergoing various stressors. This has been reported by Sigg et al. (1978) in rafs undergoing restraint stress, and in rats exposed to intermittent electric shock treatment (Leenen & Shapiro, 1974), in rats undergoing neurogenic stress, induced by crowding (Markov et al., 1976),

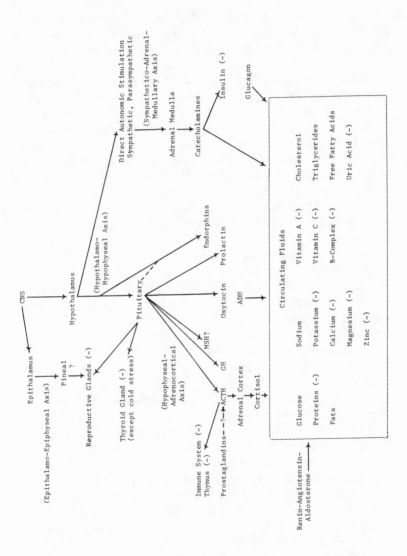

Figure 22

Factors that stimulate the secretion of renin, angiotensin, and aldosterone.

and in rats exposed to immobilization stress (Jindra, Jr. & Kvetnansky, 1982). Still other researchers have found renin secretion to
be enhanced in monkeys exposed to a psychological stimulus (Blair
et al., 1976).

Tsukiyama et al. (1973) studied the effects of the renin-angiotensin system and the pituitary-adrenocortical system in male rabbits
exposed to immobilization stress. These researchers reported a
marked increase in arterial pressure, a significant increase in plasma
renin levels and plasma corticosterone concentrations, shortly after
the onset of immobilization stress. They stated that the changes in
plasma renin did not, throughout the period of the applied immobilization stress, coincide with the plasma corticosterone concentrations. These researchers concluded that different mechanisms
activate the renin-angiotensin system and the pituitary-adrenocortical system.

Circulating renin levels were also studied in human subjects exposed to different types of stressors. The research work reported by
Wernze et al. (1975) demonstrated that plasma renin activity increased significantly in patients undergoing ear operations during
halothane anesthesia, whereas surgical manipulations had no
further influence on renin activity.

Januszewicz et al. (1979) reported that in healthy subjects, and
patients with essential hypertension, who were given a mental
stress test, the plasma renin activity increased significantly in both
groups. However, these researchers found the increase to be more
pronounced in healthy subjects.

Kosunen et al. (1976) studied plasma renin activity, angiotensin
II, and aldosterone, in male students subject to heat stress (sauna).
These researchers observed increased plasma renin activity, increased levels of angiotensin II, and increased aldosterone levels,
both during and after the sauna. They reported that the greater
mean increases in plasma renin activity were observed at the end of
the period of heat stress. They concluded that intense heat stress in
normal healthy subjects can result in large changes in the three
components of the renin-angiotensin-aldosterone system.

Syvalahti et al. (1976) studied the effect of psychic stress on
healthy medical students who were subject to an oral and written

examination. These researchers studied the release of GH, insulin, and plasma renin activity. They reported that GH, insulin, and plasma renin activity all rose after both a written and oral examination, although the mean values of renin were within the normal range of an upright posture. They reported that the levels of plasma renin activity did not appear to be a function of the duration of the examination period.

Effect of Stress on Kidney Function

Kountz (1975) studied the effects of acute stress on renal function in healthy donors. The preliminary data of this researcher suggests that, in the presence of a conflict (psychic stress), individuals may respond with an increase in blood pressure, a retention of sodium and water, and a decrease in both renal blood flow and glomerular filtration rate. Kountz further reported that if these subjects were relieved of their conflict, the above effects can be rapidly reversed.

Summary

The above-mentioned research and several other reports clearly demonstrate the response of the renin-angiotensin-aldosterone system to various types of stress exposure in both humans and animals. Clearly, most reports point to elevated levels of plasma renin activity, angiotensin, and aldosterone. These hormones contribute toward elevating blood pressure and increasing sodium and water retention by the body, typically observed in several stressful states. The underlying physiological mechanisms involved in bringing about the elevated levels in renin plasma activity during the various types of stress exposure are not completely known.

PROSTAGLANDINS

Prostaglandins (PG'S) are found distributed throughout the animal kingdom. They are prevalent in a wide variety of mammalian tissues (Samuelson et al., 1975). In fact, it is safe to say that almost every tissue of the body contains very small to moderate amounts of these substances. They were first found in humans in 1930, as a constituent of prostatic fluid, from which they derived their name. These hormones are now known to be present in almost all human tissues, and their physiological and pharmacological effects are probably just as numerous as their variety of distribution.

The activity of the prostaglandins seem to be intimately related to the activities of several other hormone and enzyme systems. Evidence to date indicates that PG's may exert some control over adenyl cyclase activity and the production of cyclic AMP. Their influence on this system may be either excitatory or inhibitory. Hence, the PG's may serve as intracellular "switches" that can turn various cellular activities on or off.

The physiological effects of the PG's are both endocrine and metabolic in nature (Bergström et al., 1968; Horton, 1969; and Ramwell & Shaw, 1970). On the pathological side, they are known to be secreted during tissue inflammation (Ferriera et al., 1975) and in the presence of noxious stimuli (Änggard and Jonsson, 1972; and Markelonis & Garbus, 1975). A wide variety of other stimuli may also influence prostaglandin release. Prostaglandin levels are increased in local tissue fluids and in the systemic circulation under both physiological and pathological conditions.

With regard to the vascular system, some prostaglandins cause vasoconstriction while others are vasodilator agents. But to date, no specific pattern of control on the vascular system has been found for the prostaglandins.

The PG's are categorized according to the degree of unsaturation and the chemical groups which are attached to the cyclic portion of the molecule. Such categorization lends itself to four distinct types of prostaglandins. The E and F groups will be mentioned here since their physiological effects have been investigated to a greater extent. Some of the physiological effects of these different types of prostaglandins include (1) PGE_1 exerts a depressive effect on gastric secretion; (2) PGE stimulates contractions of uterine smooth muscle; (3) PGF constricts and relaxes vascular smooth muscle. Hence, as mentioned previously, prostaglandins are vasodilator and some are vasoconstrictor agents; (4) PGE_2 is capable of lowering blood volume by enhancing the loss of sodium and water by the kidney. This effect can lead to a decrease in blood pressure; (5) PGF_2 has been shown to influence the production or degradation of neuro-transmitters. PGF_2 is not a neurotransmitter, but it can decrease synaptic transmission and increase neuronal rates of discharge; and (6) These ubiquitous compounds also have several effects on the circulation, but their role in circulatory control has not yet been clearly defined.

Prostaglandins and Stress

Several instances are reported in the literature in which the prostaglandins, particularly of the E series, are stimulatory to various levels of the hypothalamic-hypophyseal-adrenocortical axis. The fact that some prostaglandins are also known to stimulate ACTH secretion, both at the level of the hypothalamus (Hedge, 1976) and the anterior pituitary (Vale et al., 1971), clearly implicates them in the stress response.

Gréen and Samuelson (1971) describe experiments which demonstrate that cold stress in rats induces an increase in the synthesis and production of prostaglandins. For example, Flack et al. 1969), have shown that prostaglandins directly stimulate in vitro adrenal-cortical steroidgenesis. Vale et al. (1971) have shown that PGE can increase ACTH secretion from in vitro pituitaries. Also, Hedge and Hanson (1972), deWied, et al. (1969), and Peng et al. (1970), demonstrated that prostaglandin E, at low concentrations, when injected into the tall veins of rats, can stimulate the hypothalamic-hypophyseal-adrenal cortical axis. In particular, Hedge and Hanson (1972) indicate that the E_1, F_{1a}, and F_2 prostaglandins are capable of stimulating the secretion of ACTH, at least indirectly, by exerting an influence on the median eminence of the hypothalamus, presumably through the release of corticotropin releasing hormone. These researchers also reported that the PGF_{1a} prostaglandin appeared to be less potent than the PGE_1 prostaglandin in mediating the above effects. This variation in potency could very well reflect the fact that PGF_{1a} is more rapidly degraded in the blood than PGE_1.

DeWied et al., (1969) demonstrated that certain prostaglandins could enhance ACTH secretion in several assay systems commonly used for corticotropin-releasing hormone assays. Also, Peng et al. (1970) demonstrated that after iv PGE_1 injection, secretion of ACTH increased. Peng and his colleagues concluded that the effect of prostaglandins on ACTH release is an indirect one, being exerted at some level of the central nervous system. Their conclusions were based on pharmacological studies.

It is clear from the work of several researchers that the prostaglandins appear to exert an influence at the hypothalamic level in order to increase the secretion of ACTH. However, the mechanism and physiological significance of this prostaglandin activity remains to be elucidated.

Hanukoglu (1977) advanced the hypothesis that some prostaglandins may be the first mediators of the stress response according to the theory of stress as first proposed by Selye (1950, 1975). Hanukoglu proposes that Selye's stress theory can provide a basis within which some of the physiological functions of the various prostaglandins can be better integrated as well as understood. This researcher proposes that the prostaglandins may be identified as the primary mediators involved in the stress response, and if this is indeed the case, our understanding of stress and the general adaptation syndrome will be greatly enhanced. This same researcher also proposes that, although prostaglandins have a rapid metabolism and transit time through the circulatory system, it may well be that the derivatives of the prostaglandins, rather that the prostaglandins themselves, when released during stress, can influence and stimulate the hypothalamic-hypophyseal axis.

However, other researchers (Kehlet et al., 1977), in studies of prostaglandin release from traumatized peripheral tissue claim no support for the hypothesis that prostaglandins may act as first mediators of stress. These researchers claim that their results do not exclude a role for prostaglandins or even other hormones as mediators of other forms of stress.

Summary

Indeed, while much work is yet needed in order to investigate the physiological and pharmacological effects of the prostaglandins, their role in the elicitation of the stress response has certainly been implicated. The possible influence of the prostaglandins at the level of the cAMP mechanism and the evidence available, which indicates their stimulatory effects on ACTH secretion, clearly places them in a key position, when viewed from the perspective of stressology. However, as indicated, further research is needed in order to clarify their regulatory role, and their function as hormonal mediators involved in stress responsivity.

ENDOGENOUS OPIATES

"Endorphin" is the name given to a class of substances which have emerged from discoveries made through recent research in the field of brain opiate receptors and endogenous opiate-like peptides. Opiates have been quite popular and have been in clinical use for centuries. They are distinguished for their sedative and calming effects. However, many opiates have addictive properties, and the search for nonaddictive opiates has been in progress for several years. The recent discovery of the endorphins, which seem to be found in those areas of the brain and spinal cord which are concerned with pain perception, have opiate-like activity, and may very well prove to fit this role. The endorphins are "morphine-like" peptides and, like the pharmacological opioids, produce analgesia and catatonia.

The endorphins are synthesized in several tissues, most notably in the gastrointestinal tract, the pituitary, and the central nervous system. They are found in both the central and somatic divisions of the nervous system. Endorphin activity has been found in practically all areas of the brain. These substances function as both neurotransmitters and neuromodulators, and may play a role in the regulation of both neural and endocrine functions.

Most of the known endorphins are structured in the form of small peptides. Their amino acid sequences form part of a larger anterior pituitary peptide hormone, called β-lipotropin. The name "enkephalin" has been given to two pentapeptides, as a special type of brain endorphin. Enkephalins are found in the brains of all vertebrates studied. These substances are found in the medulla, pons, and spinal cord and even higher quantities of them are found in the hypothalamus, and limbic regions. As described in Chapter 2, these brain regions are involved in the expression of emotion, and occupy a key position in the elicitation of the stress response.

Endogenous Opiates and Stress

Recent reports indicate that β-endorphin is secreted in response to stress (Rossier et al., 1977, and Guillemin et al., 1977). More interestingly, it has been shown that β-endorphin and the anterior polypeptide hormone adrenocorticotropin, ACTH, are secreted concomitantly, in almost equimolar amounts, as a result of the elicitation of the stress response (Guillemin et. al., 1977). It should be noted that structural relationships exist between the two different polypeptides (Guillemin et al., 1977, and Mains et al., 1977). Amir et al. (1979) also present evidence that the endorphins may play a role in stress, and may be linked to the secretion of ACTH.

Recent research also indicates that the endorphins may be involved in animal learning and behavior (Riley et al., 1980). These researchers describe several models in which the endorphins were shown clearly to influence learning. In other words, in learning paradigms involving stress, these researchers demonstrated that the stressor elicits the secretion of endorphins. Also, in stress-induced analgesia, it was observed that the stress-induced release of endorphins modulated the aversiveness of the stressor and, as such, the learning based on the stressor was affected. Further evidence also points to the fact that the endorphins may play a role in the process of adaptive behavior (Verebey et al., 1978; Kosterlitz, 1979; North, 1979; and Barchas et al., 1978) and in rather selective behavioral processes under specific conditions (Abrams et al., 1978; Hayes et al., 1978; and Wesche & Frederickson, 1979). Amir et al. (1979) also studied the role of endorphins in stress and suggest that they may play a role in the behavioral concomitants of stress. These researchers suggest that the endorphins may function as modulators of neural systems that mediate the elaboration and expression of the reactive/affective components of stress.

Other types of stress have been shown to enhance plasma endorphin levels. Cohen et al. (1981) present data to suggest that surgical stress in humans may increase the plasma β-endorphin levels. Rossier et al. (1977) demonstrated that foot-shock induced stress promotes about a five- to sixfold increase in β-endorphin plasma levels. These same researchers also present data which suggest that the increases in plasma β-endorphin levels, induced by stress, do not result in elevated levels of brain β-endorphin.

Rossier et al. (1980) studied the release of prolactin induced by stress. These researchers reported that under certain experimental conditions, the blood levels of these two pituitary hormones, prolactin and β-endorphin, varied synchronously. These researchers concluded from their studies that stress exposure from footshocks, or morphine, increased the blood levels of both β-endorphin and prolactin. Also, dexamethasone (a synthetic ACTH inhibitor) pretreatment abolished the β-endorphin and prolactin response to stress. Other researchers have also found the endorphins to play a role in the stress-induced release of prolactin (Grandison & Guidotti, 1977, and Harms et al., 1975). Interestingly, Harms et al. (1975) also demonstrated parallel changes in secretion of ACTH and prolactin, induced by stress. These researchers propose that a common mechanism may be involved in the release of these hormones. This is to be viewed in terms of the work of Rossier et al. (1977) which suggest that during stress, β-endorphin is secreted by the pituitary gland.

Evidence is also available which indicates that the endogenous opioid peptides may play a role in the pathogenesis of stress hyperglycemia (Ipp et al., 1980b). An involvement of the endogenous opioids in the process of glucoregulation is presented by Amir and Bernstein (1981). These researchers exposed mice to the stress of intermittent inescapable foot shock for one hour and found the presence of a significant hyperglycemia. They demonstrated that pretreatment with a long-lasting narcotic antagonist prevented stress hyperglycemia. This same narcotic antagonist did not affect blood glucose in unstressed mice. These researchers suggest an involvement of the endogenous opioids in the stress-induced hyperglycemic response in mice.

The endorphins may also influence the pancreas by enhancing glucagon secretion (Ipp et al., 1980a, b; Ipp et al., 1978; and Kauter et al., 1980). They do not seem to be significantly involved in insulin secretion in vivo (Tannenbaum et al., 1979) nor in the inhibition of insulin during stress (Porte & Robertson, 1973; and Woods & Porte, 1974). In conditions of stress, or even of diabetes mellitus, insulin secretion is depressed. Here, the endogenous opioids may contribute toward glucagon and/or catecholamine-induced hyperglycemia (Woods & Porte, 1974).

The endorphins have also been implicated in the phenomenon of analgesia. Recently, it has been shown that analgesia can be induced by several types of stressors (Akil et al., 1976; Sherman et al., 1981; and Belenky et al., 1981). The involvement of the opioid and non-opioid mechanism in the development of stress analgesia was studied by some researchers (Lewis et al., 1980; and Lewis et al., 1982). These researchers suggest that both opioid and non-opioid mechanisms are involved in stress analgesia. They further suggest that it is possible for opiate receptors themselves to be modified by chronic stress.

Summary

It has been demonstrated by several researchers that the endogenous opioids, the endorphins, are clearly implicated in the stress response. Their relationship to the pituitary gland and ACTH secretion has been indicated. The contribution of the endorphins to the release of other stress hormones such as prolactin and glucagon and to the development and/or enhancement of stress hyperglycemia, has also been demonstrated. The mechanisms by which the endogenous opiates contribute toward stress hyperglycemia is not at present known. The development of stress analgesia was also discussed and may involve the presence, at least in part, of the endogenous opioids.

In summary, it is believed that the endorphins are clearly of importance in further elucidating the role of the endogenous opioid (endorphin) pathways in the stress–induced changes involving several processes, some of which include pain perception, analgesia, endocrine function, and behavior.

CHAPTER 14

Measurement of the Stress Response

Stress reactivity within the body can be detected by measuring certain physiological end-organ responses which are a result of sympathetic activation. Such end-organ responses include heart rate, breathing rate, and the measurement of blood pressure. Elevation above normal of any one or any combination of these parameters is an indication of sympathetic arousal and/or heightened adrenal medullary activity.

Determination of the presence of circulating stress hormones, as indicators of adrenal medullary and cortical activity, is also in wide use as a measure of the stress response. Blood and urinary levels of the catecholamines, epinephrine and norepinephrine, as well as the corticosteroids, can be measured. In this section, two categories of measurements of the stress response are described, namely, chemical and physiological measurements.

PLASMA LEVELS OF CATECHOLAMINES IN ADULTS (ng/ml)		
	NORMAL	SEVERE STRESS
EPINEPHRINE	0.05	0.27
NOREPINEPHRINE	0.20	4.10

Table III
Plasma Levels of Catecholamines in Adults.

CHEMICAL MEASUREMENTS

Catecholamines

Epinephrine and norepinephrine can be measured in blood samples by several techniques, many of which depend on fluorescence measurements or on the conversion of radioactive-labeled catecholamines to familiar end-products (radioimmune assay methods). Typical plasma levels of catecholamines, under normal and stressed conditions, are shown in Table III. It must be remembered that the blood levels of these hormones vary widely, and are a function of the state of the subject being tested.

As can be seen from Table **III**, the concentration of norepinephrine in the blood, under normal conditions, is approximately four times the level of epinephrine (Engelman & Portnoy, 1970; and Williams, 1981). Plasma values of these catecholamines vary from

AVERAGE 24-HOUR URINARY CATECHOLAMINE LEVELS IN ADULTS (μg)		
	NORMAL	STRESS
EPINEPHRINE	2-51	> 51
NOREPINEPHRINE	25-50	> 50

Table IV
Average 24-Hour Urinary Catecholamine Levels in Adults.

laboratory to laboratory, and depend on the test conditions. Tietz (1976) reports plasma levels (mean values) for epinephrine as 0.22 ng/ml and for norepinephrine as 0.58 ng/ml under normal conditions.

Twenty-four hour urine samples of the catecholamines are also measured in many clinical laboratories. Typical values for total urinary catecholamines range from 0 - 100 μg/24 hour sample under normal test conditions in different subjects (in various states of stress and nonstress). Under psychological stress, the catecholamine excretion, as detected in urine samples, can increase to levels of catecholamine producing tumors (pheochromocytoma). Catecholamine excretions, under these conditions, can approach values close to and greater than 300 μg per day (Williams, 1981). Table IV list the average values of urinary catecholamines in a 24-hour sample under normal conditions (Goodman & Gilman, 1980), and during stress.

17-Hydroxycorticosteroids in Adults		
	Plasma (μg/100ml)	Urine (μg/24 hr. sample)
Normal 8:00 a.m.	6.5-26.3	20-100
4:00 p.m.	2.0-18.0	
Stress	> 26	> 100

Table V
17-Hydroxycorticosteroids in Adults.

The 17-Hydroxycorticosteroids

Determination of the corticosteroids (adrenal cortical hormones) can be fairly accurately assessed. Cortisol, the most active adrenal cortical hormone in humans is secreted at an average rate of 20 mg/day (Guyton, 1981). Blood concentration of cortisol fluctuates diurnally and averages 12 μg percent (Guyton, 1981). A group of urinary metabolites of cortisol can be used to estimate the daily cortisol excretion rates. These are the 17-hydroxycorticosteroids (17-OHCS). These values are also subject to natural diurnal fluctuations. Table V presents a typical range of values for the 17-OHCS in plasma (Tietz, 1976), and in urinary samples (Tepperman, 1975), under normal conditions in adults. During stress, the levels of these metabolites exceed the normal range.

It should be kept in mind that the actual values obtained in any test measurement are a function of the physiological state of the subject, the adequacy of the sample collection, the means of assay, the test conditions, and the manner in which the procedure is performed.

OTHER PHYSIOLOGICAL MEASUREMENTS
OF THE STRESS RESPONSE

Recently, the field of Biofeedback has emerged and has established its place in the arena of clinical medicine. It offers the client the opportunity to be an active participant in the maintenance of his/her own health. Biofeedback involves the use of specialized instrumentation which feeds back to the client data on psychophysiological processes which the subject may not normally be aware of. The elicitation of the stress response can be mirrored through these processes, and can be easily detected with biofeedback instrumentation. It it the complex interrelationships and interactions of the cognitive, affective, and physical components which are at the core of much of biofeedback training. The major psychophysiological processes that are used in biofeedback training, and which are available to assess levels of stress reactivity within the individual are described below.

Electromyography

It is well known that many individuals respond to anxiety and other stressful conditions by tensing their muscles. It was the pioneer work of Edmund Jacobson (1938) which first showed that skeletal muscle tension and arousal states are highly correlated in a positive way. The levels of skeletal muscle tension can be measured by means of an electromyograph (EMG). Sensors placed on the skin surface can detect the electrical activity which occurs in the various underlying muscle groups. The greater the electrical activity, the higher are the measured levels of tension in the muscle group. The type of condition which is being treated with biofeedback will determine the site of EMG measurement and training. The use of EMG biofeedback has been useful in the treatment of several stress-related disorders such as tension headaches and muscular spasms. Electromyography, with or without feedback, offers a means whereby stress reactivity resulting in elevated muscle tension levels can be assessed.

Temperature Measurements and Plethysmography

Information on vascular tone can be obtained by measuring the temperature on the surface of the skin, as in temperature biofeedback, or, using plethysmographic techniques, by obtaining measurements on blood volume changes. Arousal, due to sympathetic discharge, and heightened adrenal medullary norepinephrine activity, leads to constriction of the peripheral blood vessels. This in turn leads to changes in peripheral blood flow. These changes can be easily detected by skin surface temperature measurements. Actually, minute changes in skin temperature can be assessed by the placement of thermistors on the skin surface of any portion of the limbs of the body. These include the fingers, hands, forearms, toes, and calves which are also the most common areas to measure blood volume changes through plethysmography. It is in these regions that most individuals react with a decrease in blood volume during the elicitation of the stress response. Temperature feedback has been successfully applied in the treatment of many stress-related disorders such as migraine headaches and Raynaud's syndrome. Measurements of peripheral temperture and/or blood volume serve as another tool to assess stress reactivity.

Cardiovascular Activity

Measurements of blood pressure as well as heart rate are other psychophysiological processes which can be easily and accurately assessed. During the stress response, secretion of adrenal medullary epinephrine is increased and exerts its influence on the heart. Either plethysmographic techniques or the electrocardiogram (EKG) are used to assess heart rate.

Electrodermal Measurement

States of arousal, due primarily to sympathetic nervous system discharges are measured by the galvanic skin response (GSR). Other approaches measure skin potential (SP) and electrodermal response (EDR). Basically, various states of arousal induce changes in perspiration, and this alters the electrical resistance and conductivity on the surface of the skin. This alteration in electrical activity acts as an indicator of the stress response. When used in biofeedback, individuals can receive information on their own arousal levels. These measurements, with or without feedback, offer the clinician another approach to assess states of arousal as a result of the elicitation of the stress response.

Electroencephalography

Another and less used measurement of the stress response which measures brain wave patterns, is an electroencephalograph (EEG). Measurements of electrical activity at the cortical level of the brain are converted into particular brain wave frequencies and amplitudes, which constitute the EEG. It is observed that different subjective experiences correspond with different frequencies. Attentiveness, anxiousness, or arousal correspond with beta frequencies (14 Hz and above). Meditative and passive perceptions correspond with alpha frequencies (8–13 Hz). Passive problem solving is associated with theta frequencies (4–7 Hz) and finally, the delta frequencies (3 Hz or lower) form a normal component of sleep patterns of all ages. The stress response is associated with certain subjective states tending more toward arousal and alertness. In this respect, the EEG can serve a role in assessing the levels of stress in the body. EEG biofeedback is useful in treating certain kinds of stress-related disorders including some depression states, pain, and insomnia.

SUMMARY

The above discussion has presented some available and practical chemical and physiological methods to assess stress reactivity within the organism. However, no objective device is available today which can fully measure the intensity of a stressor and its subsequent influence on end-organ responsivity within the organism.

Various psychological tools also exist to assess the stress response. These tools are numerous and focus on measurements of various psychological components of the organism. The psychological assessment is then evaluated in terms of the stress response. In this chapter, we have briefly focused on the chemical and physiological determinations of the stress response, and have not entered into a discussion concerning the procedures for psychological assessment. It is not the scope of this text to discuss such psychological measurements of the stress response, but it is necessary to emphasize that these tools are indeed important and should form an integral part of the total assessment procedure. Due to the multifactorial nature of stress reactivity, an integrative approach, which takes into account several indicators of measurement, is needed. This is necessary in order accurately to assess the degree of psychophysiological arousal within the organism.

CHAPTER 15

Stress and Disease

THE LINK BETWEEN STRESS AND DISEASE

Chronic elecitation of the stress response ultimately leads to end-organ dysfunction. But the means whereby a specific end-organ dysfunction emerges as a result of the stress response, is not presently known. It is, however, known that all the stress response pathways discussed in previous chapters cannot be activated simultaneously within the same subject and remain activated, nor can every end-organ be influenced within the same individual to the same degree of intensity during the stress response.

Various theories have emerged to discuss the relationship between psychophysiological arousal, individual differences, and specific end-organ dysfunction. While many of these theories contribute to our understanding of these relationships, no one theory to date has been able to provide a direct link between psychophysiological arousal, individual differences and specific end-organ pathology. However, it is commonly accepted that the means by which a particular end-organ develops pathological or dysfunctional symptomology, is related to the chronicity of the psychophysiological arousal state and the hyperstimulation of the specific end-organ. The outcome of such a state is the development of a disease or stress-related disorder (specific end-organ dysfunction), over a period of time, as a result of persistent hyperarousal reactivity patterns, that is, from frequent to prolonged overstimulation. Also, several factors such as genetic predisposition, lifestyle habits, etc. are thought to contribute to the variation in individual differences known to occur in the development of stress-related disorders. A brief description of some commonly encountered stress-related disorders prevalent in our society today, along with a description of their neurophysiological pathways of development are discussed below.

NEUROPHYSIOLOGICAL PATHWAYS OF STRESS-RELATED DISORDERS

Chronic stress reactivity may activate one or more different neurophysiological pathways which, in the long term, can result in end-organ dysfunction. There are probably several neurophysiological pathways which relate to end-organ symptomology developed because of stress exhaustion. Four of these neurophysiological pathways have been described and categorized, for the purpose of arriving at a better understanding of the diagnosis, prognosis, and treatment, of stress-related disorders (Wilson & Schneider, 1981). These same authors claim that this categorization may also open the way to further elucidate the underlying mechanisms involved in the genesis of end-organ pathology as a result of chronic hyperarousal states. A description of these four neurophysiological pathways as described by Wilson and Schneider is given below.

Interneuronal Stress Response

The central and peripheral nervous system may be the predominant axis through which adaptation to distress may occur. Adaptation to chronic stress leading to distress may manifest itself in a progressive change (increase, decrease, or change in composition) of neurotransmitters both within the central and peripheral nervous systems. Both endogenous and exogenous pathways for neuro-transmitter alteration appear to exist.

"Endogenous pathways of neurotransmitter aberrations may have a familial/congenital origin such as manic depressive disease, schizophrenia or endogenous depression. These disorders seem to involve a decrease in biogenic amines in the case of depression, and an increase in the case of mania. Schizophrenia may also involve an abnormal excess of dopamine." (Wilson & Schneider, 1981).

Peripheral nervous system dysfunction, which results from alterations of neurotransmitter substances, may include such disorders as multiple sclerosis and myasthenia gravis. Factors, other than neurotransmitter alterations, may be involved. For example, considering the case of myasthenia gravis, evidence is available, to indicate, that it may be an autoimmune disease. Whatever the combination of factors involved, these end-stage diseases may be a product of chronic overstimulation of neuronal pathways resulting in abnormal alterations in neurotransmitter substances and neuro-transmitter release.

Normal functioning of neurotransmitter activity may also be interferred with through the habitual use of pharmacological agents. These typify the exogenous interneuronal pathways of adaptation to chronic stress. The drugs or chemicals in question include many which have become popular today as part of one's coping strategies or reactive behavior patterns to chronic stress. Examples include the use of caffeinated beverages, nicotine, and various "uppers" and "downers." The side effects produced by these substances, can, in the long term result in physiological end-organ dysfunction. Chronic use of any drug or chemical can result in unpleasant side-effects and altered physiology with changes in normal adaptive mechanisms.

Neurovascular Stress Response

Vascular manifestations of the "fight or flight" response have been described earlier. As mentioned previously, distress or end-organ dysfunction can occur as a result of the accumulation of many unresolved "fight or flight" responses. The notable changes include a shunting of blood away from the periphery resulting in peripheral vasoconstriction, positive ionotropic and chronotropic effects on the heart, and an elevation in blood pressure. If intense enough, diastolic pressure may also increase resulting in an elevation in pulse pressure. All these changes while acute and intermittent at first, may then become chronic in later stages. This can pave the way for the many cardiovascular disorders that are most popular in this country today, particularly, hypertension. Also, the intense elevations in blood pressure that initially occur may also result in a slow tearing away of coronary artery tissue. Many such insults could result in the deposition of fibrin and cholesterol in blood vessel walls leading to coronary artery occlusion.

Other vascular disorders resulting from extending the chronic elicitation of the stress response to the end stage of distress include severe migraine headaches, Raynaud's syndrome, and severe menstrual cramps. Also, increased vagal tone and elevated levels of stress hormones coupled with the chronic vascular response to stress have been seen in subjects suffering from various cardiac arrhythmias and paroxysmal arterial tachycardia.

In summary, the chronic elicitation of the vascular stress response can lead to coronary artery disease, other vascular disorders and major heart disease even in the absence of the commonly known risk factors.

Vascular responders to chronic stress show immediate decreases in digital hand temperature when placed under stress. Biofeedback, utilizing the modality of temperature training has been shown to provide a useful method for vascular responders to develop inner controls, thereby aiding in the cultivation and maintenance of lowered arousal states.

Neuromuscular Stress Response

The skeletal muscular system performs its mechanical activity of contraction followed by relaxation through the process of electrical excitation from neuronal inputs. Microscopically, neural innervation of muscle fibers occurs at the neuromuscular junction, in a region called the end-plate. Here, neurotransmitter release from nerve endings alters the ionic events taking place at the membrane level of the muscle fibers. This results in the contraction of muscle fibers. The events taking place are referred to as electrosecretory coupling (release of the neurotransmitter substance, acetylcholine, by nerve endings) followed by excitation-contraction coupling (excitation of the muscle membranes leading to the mechanical event of contraction).

As the nervous system becomes more and more involved in hyperstimulated activity, the muscles slowly but surely fail to return to a resting state or baseline level after each tonic contraction. The result is a gradual escalation in muscle contraction or tension. As the tension in the muscle increases over a period of time, there is a gradual development of metabolic waste products in the intercellular spaces surrounding the muscle fibers, and in the muscle fibers themselves. This is a result of poor drainage due to prolonged contraction of veins and lymphatics caused by the build-up of tension. This altered biochemical and physiological state of the muscle results in continued contractions even without added electrical activity from innervating neurons. These conditions may very well be the predisposing factors which result in the familiar aches and pains experienced during the build-up of muscular tension, (Wilson and Schneider, 1981).

Common muscular dysfunction resulting from chronic elicitation of the stress response includes such conditions as tension headaches, lower back pain, muscle spasms in the neck and shoulder areas, and spasm of various other muscle groups in the body.

Skeletal muscle spasm may lead to end-organ pathophysiology which include diseases such as fibrosis, and several degenerative joint diseases.

Muscle responders to chronic stress can be treated effectively with EMG biofeedback training, provided that the above-mentioned end-stage pathophysiology of the muscular system is not present. Progressive muscle relaxation and other deep muscle relaxation methods, have also been shown to be effective modalities of treatment.

Neurohumoral Stress Response

Chronic elicitation of the stress response results in prolonged activation of the neuroendocrine pathways or axes, discussed previously in the text. A number of stress hormones may become prevalent in the circulation. Among the most common hormones discussed in the text include elevated levels of ACTH and cortisol, epinephrine and norepinephrine. All of these hormones at higher concentrations, exert specific physiological effects, many of which were discussed in the text. For example, under the influence of cortisol, the immune system is depressed. This may be mediated by the cortisol-induced atrophy of the thymolymphatic system. Also several studies presently underway indicate that individuals undergoing major life changes, are more susceptible to infection, and show a higher incidence of certain tumor (leukemia, lymphoma, etc.) development. Again, the implication for stress-induced immunosuppressive activity is indicated.

From the text, the hypothalamus was described as a crucial structure in the expression of the stress response. It stands in a hierarchical position of control to regulate and mediate autonomic nervous system activation, various endocrine gland functions and certain basic physiological processes. In addition to autonomic nervous system regulation, and the regulation of secretion of several pituitary hormones as described in the text, the hypothalamus is also involved in the regulation of such processes as thirst, appetite, body temperature, pleasure and pain. Due to the position the hypothalamus holds in mediating the stress response, any functions which come under hypothalamic control may also be altered during stress. For example, eating patterns may change during chronic stress. Some persons may gain weight and others may lose weight—both patterns can potentially lead to several disease states and end-organ dysfunction. The mechanisms by which these changes occur are not well understood. Also, as discussed at length in the text, other endocrine axes may be affected by stress, such as the thyroid and the reproductive axes.

For example, during cold stress, the thyroid gland is activated because of the stress-induced secretion of TSH. Hence, all the processes of the body are accelerated. Other types of stress exposure, on the other hand, appear to suppress thyroid gland activity.

The gonadotropin hormones, LH and possibly FSH, may be suppressed during chronic stress. In the female, this results in decreased levels of estrogen and progesterone. The sexual cycle is disrupted, and conditions such as amennorhea may develop. In the male, testosterone secretion appears to be decreased as a result of various types of stress exposure. Four neurophysiological pathways which may be activated by chronic stress reactivity and which can lead in the long term to end-organ dysfunction have been briefly described. Other neurophysiological pathways undoubtedly exist.

Since an assessment of the degree of reactivity along any one of these four stress response pathways cannot be made directly, a number of strategies and techniques have emerged which focus on reduction of symptomology. Stress reduction training including deep breathing exercises, deep muscle relaxation, biofeedback, and several other methods, focus on the cultivation of low arousal states, with a primary goal oriented toward maintaining these states. For a more comprehensive treatment of this topic, the reader is again referred to the work of Wilson and Schneider (1981).

STRESS MANAGEMENT STRATEGIES

Stress management strategies can be applied to the four pathways of the stress response described above, with their attendant symptomology, in order to alter the course of physiological changes which occur during the chronic elicitation of the stress response. In other words, these methods are helpful when applied prior to the onset of end-organ pathophysiology. Several stress-management strategies have been adequately described in various professional and popular texts. However, for the sake of completion, some of these methods will be summarized below.

Many strategies and combinations of strategies are in use today for particular treatment purposes. These stress-management strategies are a function of many factors, some of which include the type of response to be altered, and the reactivity patterns of the client. a prerequisite to training, recognition of client symptoms and patterns of distress must be adequately assessed.

Interneuronal Stress Response

The response patterns associated with this state of distress revolve around the symptoms of altered cognitions and emotions such as fear and/or depressions. Hence, treatment strategies should include cognitive restructuring methods. Biofeedback procedures which train for lowered arousal states may be employed as an adjunctive modality of treatment. The methods of systematic desensitization, positive covert sensitization, and rational emotive training, are also beneficial in treating this type of stress response pattern.

Neurovascular Stress Response

Cardiovascular responders to stress, such as the coronary prone Type A personality, can benefit from different modalities of biofeedback training. Depending on the symptomology present, heart rate, blood pressure and temperature training have been shown to be beneficial. GSR training for lowered arousal levels can be a helpful adjunctive modality. Some of these methods were briefly alluded to in the previous chapter. Techniques which induce physiological relaxation such as autogenic training, the quieting response, meditation and the use of imagery have also been shown to be useful adjunctive therapies.

Neuromuscular Stress Response

As mentioned in the previous chapter, muscle tension developed as a result of the chronic elicitation of the stress response, can be treated successfully with EMG biofeedback. Generalized relaxation training utilizing frontalis muscle tension reduction and/or relaxation training for particular muscle groups of the body generally comprise a treatment program utilizing EMG biofeedback. Other relaxation training exercises such as deep muscle relaxation, progressive muscle relaxation, visual imagery and techniques adapted from yogic principles, have been shown to be helpful.

Neurohumoral Stress Response

At least at present, this pathway is not amendable to direct biofeedback training as such. The various hormonal secretions and levels of hormones and other metabolites in the blood may best be influenced by general relaxation methods which include meditative and imagery type of techniques.

For a more comprehensive treatment of this topic, and the topic of stress related disorders the reader is referred to Everly, Jr. and Rosenfeld, 1981; Girdano and Everly, 1979; and Wilson and Schneider, 1981.

STRESS-RELATED DISORDERS

Stress has been strongly linked to disease (Cassel, 1970; Holme & Rahe, 1967; Wolff, 1953; and Selye, 1956).

It is important to emphasize that stress-related disorders develop because of chronic elicitation of the stress response. The focal point is chronic or prolonged over-reactivity. An acute response is not nearly so harmful to the body as are slight or moderate responses sustained over a prolonged time period.

According to the model proposed by Selye (1956), and as previously described in the text, distress or end-organ pathology may be experienced as a result of reaching the stress exhaustion phase. For example, the cummulative result of many unresolved "fight or flight" responses can, in the long term, progress to specific end-organ dysfunctioning. End-organ pathophysiology may become manifest and result in overt disease and possibly even death. The development of disease as a result of prolonged chronic stress on the various systems of the body is described below.

Skeletal Muscle System

Muscle comprises the greatest mass in the body and is responsible for almost every mode of bodily expression, from gross bodily movements to the fine movements involved in speech and facial expressions. This system is important during the "fight or flight" response since it enables the organism to prepare and handle a threatening situation. In this situation, the muscles increase in tone and become more tense.

Stress-related disorders develop when the tension in the muscles persist for long periods of time with little or no relief. The stress response is extended into its chronic phase. Chronically tense muscles can produce a variety of disorders such as backache, lower back pain, headache, asthma, lockjaw, esophageal and colonic spasms, arthritis and perhaps even rheumatoid arthritis.

Arthritis is a condition of inflammation of the joints and can occur as a result of infection, injury, or prolonged wear and tear on the various tissues of the body. Rheumatoid arthritis is a disease that occurs in individuals, usually in the prime of life, and may affect not only joints, but also the whole body. The diseases of arthritis may be characterized by several causal mechanisms—one of which may be a deficient functioning of the immune system. Today, several research studies indicate that stress may exert a marked influence on immunological mechanisms. Chronic stress may, therefore, be one of several components contributing to the etiology of these disease states.

Gastrointestinal System

It has been accepted over the past several years that gastrointestinal disorders are intricately tied into the psychological and emotional components of the organism and are therefore related to psychophysiological arousal states. Functional gastrointestinal disorders are frequently associated with symptoms of emotional problems and disturbances such as anxiety. Stress has been strongly implicated in disorders of the gastrointestinal tract, an example being gastric ulceration (Weiss et al., 1970; and Akiskal & McKinney, 1975). In view of the fact that the GI system serves no function in the "fight or flight" response, one may inquire as to the wide prevalence of GI disorders found in our society today. Clearly the answer must lie in the ease of responsiveness of the GI system to psychological and emotional reactivity. It may very well be that almost every structure of the GI tract responds to stress. Some examples of GI stress responsivity include: dry mouth, muscle spasms of the esophagus, stomach and colon, and disruption of peristaltic movement in both the small and large intestines. Other gastrointestinal symptoms include heart burn, cramps, bloating, abdominal rumbling and epigastric pain.

Two serious gastrointestinal disorders linked to stress over-reactivity include peptic ulcers and ulcerative colitis.

Peptic ulcers come about because of an erosion of the wall of the stomach caused by increased acid and enzyme secretions. It is known that emotions such as anger, for example, can result in gastric acid hypersecretion and can exacerbate an already existing ulcer. The etiology of this disorder is not clearly understood. Perhaps stress-induced heightened glucocorticoid anti-inflammatory activity or vagus stimulated gastric hypersecretion may play a role.

Other stress-related disorders, which occur lower in the alimentary canal, include colonic disturbances such as irritable bowel. This condition makes the individual prone to either constipation or diarrhea. The extreme of this state is ulcerative colitis where the bowel movements are impacted with blood and may become uncontrollable.

Ulcerative colitis is an inflammation of the colon lining. This condition is observed to respond to the emotional state of the individual. For example, emotions such as anger seem to precipitate this condition or exacerbate an already existing one. The etiology of the disease is not known but perhaps may be related to the stress-related increase in levels of lysozyme which dissolves the mucus in the lining of the colon. Several other factors, such as the activity of the immunological system, may contribute to the onset of this disorder.

Other Digestive Disorders

Another widespread disorder is diabetes. Evidence is mounting that this disorder is related to stress. In situations perceived as a threat, from marital or work-related confrontations to physical endurance, it has been repeatedly shown that the sugar levels in the blood rise. Psychophysiological overreactivity appears to result initially in a hyperglycemic response. Perhaps in time, this may place a burden on the pancreas. In the long term, pancreatic dysfunction may result leading to insulin deficiency.

Respiratory System

Hyperventilation: This is an effort by the organism, as part of the "fight or flight" response, to increase oxygen intake and decrease carbon dioxide elimination. It occurs as an acute response to stress.

Allergy: This is a hypersensitivity reaction where the body responds with an exaggerated defense mechanism to a particular foreign substance called an allergen. Organs that are affected in allergic reactions include those that are relatively exposed, such as, the nose, lungs, digestive tract and the skin. An allergic response, for example, to certain forms of pollen in the air result in a swelling of mucous membranes, copious nasal secretions and congestion. This is apparently an overreactivity to a particular stimulus, and is more prone to occur during stress exposure than otherwise.

Bronchial Asthma: This disorder is characterized by increased amounts of bronchial secretions and swelling of the mucosal lining. This is coupled with contractions of the smooth muscles which line the bronchioles. The result is the familiar "gasping for air" syndrome. This in itself may be stress producing and can compound the stress response produced initially. Cognitive and affective components are implicated in the onset of this pyschophysiological arousal state.

Skin Disorders

The skin with its nervous control serves as an end-organ for stress reactivity and arousal. States of arousal can be measured on the surface of the skin by two well-known parameters, namely, electrical activity and temperature. (1) The electrical conductivity of the skin surface changes as a result of the elicitation of the stress response due to the activity of heightened subdermal glandular secretions. (2) The temperature of the surface of the skin is an indicator of peripheral blood flow, which in turn, is a function of the vascular tone of the small blood vessels located under the skin. During stress and anxiety, these vessels constrict, causing a decrease in peripheral blood flow. The measured peripheral temperature then decreases. This sensitivity response pattern has been shown to serve as an indicator of prolonged psychophysiological arousal states. Some of the common stress-related disorders related to the skin include acne, eczema, urticaria, and perhaps, psoriasis. The causal mechanism involved in the genesis of these diseases is not well known, but evidence does exist to indicate that psychophysiological arousal may be one of the mediating factors.

Immune System

The body's defense against foreign invasion are handled efficiently and effectively by the immune system. This system does not function maximally at all times. Cases in point include the early years of life when the immune system is developing, and the latter years when the immune system is losing its efficiency. It has been shown that the young and the old become more susceptible to infection than the middle-age population.

There is much evidence to date to indicate that depression of the immune system occurs because of prolonged and excessive stress. Some of the pioneer work in this area was carried out by Selye (1976). In his work, he describes the immunosuppressive effect of both the adrenal cortical output of glucocorticoids and stress. The implication appears to be that if stress can indeed exert a generalized immunosuppressive effect, then it must be influential in the onset and maintenance of infectious and degenerative diseases. Today, the many pathways involved in immunosuppression are slowly and carefully being investigated.

In cancer, the immune system has failed in its function. For some reason, foreign cells live and thrive in the organism without interference. Stress may be a factor (Fox, 1978) since chronic stress appears to depress the immunological responses of the body. The question of whether it is stress in general, or whether it is a particular kind of stress that makes people cancer prone— remains to be answered. However, evidence is mounting that cancer-prone subjects are associated with distinctive states of cognitive response patterns. The implication for psychophysiological reactivity, as one component in the etiology of this diseased state, warrants continued investigation.

Cardiovascular System

Stress has been strongly linked to heart disease (Glass, 1977). Several studies have demonstrated a relationship between psychological factors and coronary heart disease (Jenkins, 1971; Friedman, 1969; and Rosenman et al., 1970).

Recent epidemiological and psychological studies strongly suggest that a certain type of behavior pattern, a coronary-prone behavior pattern, also known as the familiar Type A personality, is associated with an increased risk of coronary heart disease. Also, epidemiological research has disclosed several risk factors implicated in congestive heart disease. These risk factors include, age, sex, body weight, exercise, cholesterol, blood pressure and cigarette smoking. The most important of these thought to contribute the most impact to the genesis of coronary heart disease include, cholesterol, blood pressure, age and sex.

Disorders of the cardiovascular system focus on the heart itself, on the vasculature, on systematic blood flow, and on blood pressure. This system taken as a whole has been considered to be a major end-organ for the stress response. Dysfunction, as a result of heightened levels of stress, has produced such disorders as hypertension, arrhythmias, angina, migrane headache, and Raynaud's syndrome. The etiology of these disorders remains to be defined, yet the implication for psychophysiological arousal is present.

In hypertension, heightened activity of the sympathetic-adrenal-medullary and anterior pituitary-adrenal-cortical axes occur (Eliot, 1979). Both contribute to an elevation in blood pressure, particularly, the activity of medullary norepinephrine on the vasculature.

Stress overreactivity in the long term can also lead to the familiar cardiac disorders of arrhythmia and angina. Cardiac arrhythmia is a condition which is a direct indication that the heart is malfunctioning, but no organic damage is present, Arrhythmias of various kinds may result from stress-induced sympathetic dysfunction or vascular obstruction (Selye, 1976). Angina is a condition in which not enough oxygen supply reaches the heart. It it characterized by sharp chest pains, and perhaps feelings of suffocation. Angina may be a stress-induced condition, since anxiety and tension have often been observed to be a part of the behavior patterns of angina-prone subjects.

With regard to migraine headaches and Raynaud's syndrome, heightened sympathetic activation is strongly implicated. Migraine headaches result from cranial vasoconstriction. Cold exposure can induce vasoconstriction in the hands and feet, resulting in Raynaud's syndrome. Both of these disorders are known to be influenced by emotional distress.

It must be emphasized that although these disorders of the cardiovascular system are generally accepted to be influenced by excessive stress, the mechanism's involved in their pathophysiology remains to be elucidated. It might be added that despite variations in cardiac dysfunction, subjects with different forms of cardiac disease express a similarity in terms of personality profile, behavior patterns, and psychophysiological reactivity.

Urino-Genital System

Urinary Tract: The bladder which is under the influence of the autonomic nervous system, also appears to be affected by psychogenic-induced stimuli. It has been observed that the emotional state of fear may result in incontinence of the urine, and perhaps of even both the urine and feces. The emotional states of frustration and resentment have often been observed to be associated with bladder contraction, which results in an experience of urgency of urination. On the other hand, the emotional states of dejection appear to result in urinary retention induced by relaxation of the bladder (Staub et al., 1949).

Genital Tract: It has been observed that psychogenic-induced stimuli may influence the reproductive activity in both the male and female. Testosterone suppression in the male as well as psychogenic ammenohrea in the female as a result of various types of stress exposure, have been previously described. The process of both erection and ejaculation in the male are under autonomic nervous system influence and, as such, may be subject to psychogenic stimuli. For example, it is a well-known fact that psychological components may play a dominant role in the development of impotency.

Summary

In all of the disorders described, it must be kept in mind, that the causal mechanisms involved are multifactorial in nature. Factors such as heredity, genetic predisposition, exercise regimen, nutritional patterns, functional imbalances within the body, and lifestyle, all contribute to the development of the diseased state. As mentioned, many of the disorders described are exacerbated by intense stress. This points to the need for continued investigative work concerning the mechanisms underlying psychophysiological arousal states. Perhaps, the whole area of stress-related disorders and disease will be better understood when human psychophysiological reactivity is viewed from a more holistic or integrative perspective.

In reviewing this topic of stress-related disorders, it is relevant to consider the ideas of Hippocrates who, more than 2,300 years ago, emphasized the fact that physicians should consider the whole person (mind, emotions, as well as physical body), to diagnose and treat health-related problems properly. Hippocrates maintained that the well-being of the individual is influenced by several factors including environmental, such as the quality of the air, water, food, the topography of the land, and other factors which include general living habits.

One is also reminded of the writings of Maimonides who, over 800 years ago, stressed the point that in a very real sense, there are no illnesses but only patients. Maimonides indicated that the physician should not treat the disease but the patient who is suffering from it. In other words, according to Maimonides, it is of much greater significance to know what kind of patient has the disease than what kind of disease the patient has.

CHAPTER 16

Conclusion

The intent of this text has been to emphasize the neuroendocrine aspects or the more chronic phase of the stress response. This was accomplished through a presentation and review of the basic physiology of both the human nervous and endocrine systems, along with a review of some recent research describing the effects of various types of stressors on the different endocrine glands and their hormonal secretions in the body. Although only a limited review of the literature is presented, it is hoped that this presentation provided the reader with an understanding of the many different facets from which this subject is being approached in the experimental laboratory as well as in human test conditions. The numerous types of stressors used in the experimental paradigm, the chronicity of the applied stressor, as well as the various test conditions, all contribute toward the body of knowledge accumulated to date concerning the neuroendocrine responses to stress. The conflicting results reported on several occasions lead one to examine the nature of the stress response in terms of individual variation in perception as well as to the intensity of individual reactivity to a stressor.

It must be recalled that the body responds to the perception of a threat in a very specific way. The underlying physiological changes which occur are directed toward having the organism achieve adaptation in situations of chronic intermittent stress. This adaptation is accomplished through the effort by the organism to maintain homeostasis and to conserve its own internal energy resources.

Based on the material presented in the text, a brief summary of the neuroendocrine response to stress is shown in Figure 23 and briefly outlined below.

PHYSIOLOGY OF THE STRESS RESPONSE

Neural Axis

Peripheral and Central Nervous Systems

A stimuli induces a signal which travels to the central nervous system through nervous and/or humoral pathways.

Stress → Nervous and/or humoral pathways → Central Nervous System
↓
Brain

The signal is received by the brain where the appropriate encoding and interpretation of the signal takes place. The stimulus may also originate here as a perception in the form of a thought or an emotion.

BRAIN
(Cortex, Limbic, Reticular Activating System)

↓

Perception of a Threat

Autonomic Nervous System

The encoded signal perceived as a threat reaches the hypothalamus. The hypothalamus then sends signals along neural pathways which result in an autonomic nervous system activation (predominately sympathetic). Appropriate end-organ responses occur. This represents the first phase (neural axis) that is activated as a result of the elicitation of the stress response.

Hypothalamus → Autonomic Nervous System
↙   ↘
Sympathetic   Parasympathetic
End-Organ Response   End-Organ Response

Neuroendocrine Axis

Sympathetic-Adrenal-Medullary Axis

The next phase of stress activation involves the "fight or flight" response (sympathetic-adrenal-medullary axis). This neuroendocrine response is quite rapid, and results in the catecholamine output by the adrenal glands with its attendant physiological effects.

Sympathetic Nervous System → Adrenal Medulla ↗Epinephrine
↘Norepinephrine

Adrenal-medullary-sympathetic stimulation results in an increase of the catecholamines into the circulation. The catecholamines, in particular, epinephrine, exerts a hyperglycemic effect, that is, it causes the blood glucose levels to rise. Glycerol and free fatty acid levels are also increased in the circulation. The adrenal medullary epinephrine intensifies the phsyiological effects induced by the initial sympathetic activation. The heart rate, blood pressure, and breathing rate are increased. The blood is shunted to the muscular system, and the respiratory air passages become dilated.

The final and more chronic phase, and longest acting of all the axes activated as a result of the elicitation of the stress response, involves further stimulation of the neuroendocrine axis. The activation of this axis results in the stimulation of several different endocrine components.

Hypothalamic Posterior Pituitary Axis

By means of neurotransmitters, signals are sent to various peptidergic neurons in the hypothalamus. The hypothalamus, through nerve transmission, then activates the posterior pituitary to release its hormones, ADH and oxytocin, into the systemic circulation.

ADH

Hypothalamus → Posterior Pituitary ↗

(Supraoptic   (Neurohypophysis)
and Para-   ↘ Oxytocin
ventricular
nuclei)

Renin-Angiotensin-Aldosterone System

The renin–angiotensin–aldosterone system is activated along with ADH. Both these systems regulate the volume of fluids circulating in the body by enhancing sodium and water reabsorption by the kidneys. The catecholamines may also exert an influence on the activation of the renin-angiotensin system. During the stress response, sodium and water retention is a common phenomenon, probably mediated by the elevated levels of these hormones in the circulation.

Sympathetic Nervous System
(modulators)
Adrenal Catecholamines
ADH
Sodium
ACTH
$\downarrow$
$\rightarrow$ Renin-Angiotensin
$\downarrow$ ACTH
Aldosterone $\leftarrow$ Potassium
               Sodium
               Pineal Gland?

Glucagon and Insulin

The elevated blood glucose levels stimulate the release of glucagon from the pancreas. Glucagon enhances hepatic glycogenolysis and adds more glucose into the bloodstream. In effect, glucagon potentiates the hyperglycemic effect of the catecholamines. Simultaneously, pancreatic insulin secretion is inhibited by the catecholamines. The utilization of glucose by the peripheral tissues is therefore decreased. Glucose utilization is replaced by the release of fatty acids from adipose tissue, which in turn is used as the replacement source of energy.

Epinephrine $\rightarrow$ Blood Glucose $\leftarrow$ Glucagon
$\searrow$
Insulin $(-)$

The above description comprises the more rapid phase of activation of the neuroendocrine axis. Here the necessary stores of energy are mobilized and the vital organs involved in the stress response such as the brain, muscles, and heart, are provided with the necessary nutrients (glucose) and energy supply at the expense of the skin, kidneys, and other peripheral structures.

The next and more chronic phase of the neuroendocrine stress response involves the secretion of several other hormonal components.

The hypothalamus receiving inputs from the central nervous system is stimulated to release certain hypothalamic releasing hormones, which in turn increase the secretion of some of the anterior pituitary hormones.

The various endocrine axes and various hormones released are described below.

Anterior Pituitary-Adrenal-Cortical Axis

The hypothalamus secretes CRH, which in turn stimulates the secretion of ACTH by the anterior pituitary. MSH from the pars intermedia of the pituitary may also be secreted along with ACTH. ACTH stimulates the secretion of cortisol by the adrenal cortex. Cortisol exerts several physiological effects. The important effects of cortisol include an enhancement of the level of amino acids in the circulation and the formation of glucose from noncarbohydrate sources (gluconeogenesis). Cortisol also promotes the utilization of fats for energy. The pituitary-adrenal-cortical axis also causes a depression of the immune system. The adrenal cortical hormones are almost always stimulated as a result of the elicitation of the stress response.

$$
\begin{array}{l}
\left.\begin{array}{l} \text{MIH} \\[6pt] \text{MRH} \end{array}\right\} \rightarrow \text{MSH} \\[4pt]
\hspace{3.5em} \text{Protein Mobilization} \\
\text{CRH} \rightarrow \text{ACTH} \rightarrow \text{Cortisol} \leftrightarrows \text{Fat Mobilization} \\
\hspace{5.5em} \downarrow \hspace{3em} \text{Gluconeogenesis} \\
\hspace{4em} \text{Insulin} \,(-)
\end{array}
$$

Somatotropin Axis

Growth hormone, released by the hypothalamus, increases the secretion of somatotropin hormone, or growth hormone, by the anterior pituitary. While the release of GH is regulated by the hypothalamic releasing hormones, other hormones, such as glucagon and epinephrine, may influence its secretion. Both glucagon and GH stimulate the uptake of amino acids by cells and effect the mobilization of energy resources of the body.

$$\left.\begin{array}{c} \text{GHIH} \\ \text{GHRH} \end{array}\right\} \rightarrow \text{GH} \leftarrow \begin{array}{l} \text{Circulating levels of} \\ \text{Epinephrine and Glucagon} \end{array}$$

Other Components of the Neuroendocrine Axis

Other components of the neuroendocrine axis include the pineal gland, the endogenous opiates, and prolactin.

The epithalamo-epiphyseal-pineal axis may act to modulate the hypothalamic-hypophyseal-adrenal cortical axis during stress, through its sensitivity to sensory stimuli, and as a regulator of circadian rhythms.

Secretion of endogenous opiates increases as a result of stress and enhances the sensitivity threshold for painful stimuli. The endogenous opiates may serve in many other capacities during the stress response.

Some of the prostaglandins have also been implicated in the stress response particularly in view of their stimulatory effects on ACTH secretion.

Prolactin is increased as a result of stress. Its role in the stress response remains to be clarified.

Two endocrine axes, the thyroid and gonadotropin axis, appear to be generally suppressed as a result of the stress response.

Gonadotropin Axis

Male: Testosterone production by the testes appears to be suppressed under the influence of stress. Secretions of pituitary LH appear to be more affected by stress than FSH.

Female: The monthly cycle of hormonal secretions comprising LRH, LH, FSH, estrogen, and progesterone can be altered and the cycle diverted from its normal pattern as a result of stress. The pineal gland may exert some influence on the cycle.

Thyroid Axis

Secretion of TRH from the hypothalamus enhances the secretion of anterior pituitary TSH release, which in turn influences the hormonal output of the thyroid gland. This is true for the cold stress exposure. Other types of stress, in many cases, appear to suppress thyroid hormonal release. At this point, it appears that long-term stress exposure may depress the thyroid endocrine axis.

Several nutrients, vitamins, minerals, and other metabolic factors are known to be influenced by stress. These changes, as well as the neuroendocrine hormonal alterations, are summarized in Figure 23.

In both humans and animals, the initial components of the stress response (direct autonomic nervous system and sympathetic-adrenal-medullary stimulation) occur in the presence of almost all known types of stress exposure. The number of physiological changes which occur can be quite varied, but the essential nature of the response does not change (increased heart rate, blood pressure, etc.). However, when the more chronic neuroendocrine phase of the stress response occurs, it occurs with a greater amount of variability. Many of the endocrine components may or may not be stimulated, but when stimulated, it is with varying degrees of intensity. The hypothalamic pituitary-adrenal-cortical axis is activated in practically all cases. During chronic stress exposure, the type, severity, and chronicity of the stress exposure determines both the number and nature of the neuroendocrine response pattern. During chronic intermittent stress, or repeated exposure to the same stressor (adaptation), the hormonal responses usually attenuate to a certain degree. However, if a new and different stressor is introduced at this time, the hormonal responses will be one of increased levels of adrenal cortical hormones associated with the initial exposure to the chronic stressor. In other words, the alterations in hormonal responses are such that the maximal response usually takes place prior to the onset of the chronic phase of a stress exposure, rather than during it.

SUMMARY

The work of Cannon, in the early 1900s, incorporated the study of the changes that take place in the body as a result of various

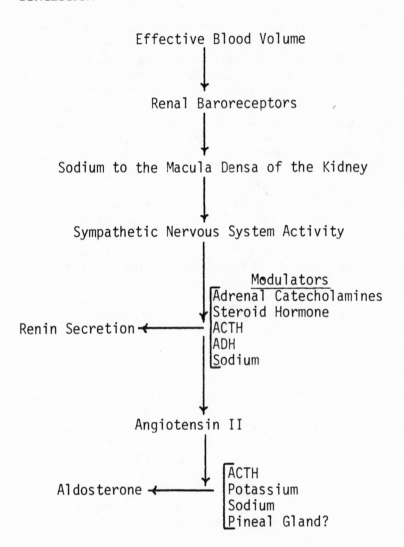

Figure 23
Suggested model of the physiology of the stress response in humans.

physical and physiological stimuli (hunger, pain), as well as various emotional states (fear, anger). He directed much of his attention to the "fight or flight" response involving the activation of the sympathetic nervous system and the adrenal medulla. His studies were primarily focused on the activity of the catecholamines.

The pioneering work of Cannon was followed by the scientific investigations of Selye, who focussed his attention on stress-related disorders and the diseases of adaptation. The work of Selye was directed primarily toward the responses of the pituitary adrenal-cortical axis, and were focused on the long-term physiological effects of the adrenal cortical hormones on the body. He discussed a triad of responses, described as adrenal cortical hypertrophy, thymicolymphatic involution, and gastrointestinal disorders, as an outcome of an alarm reaction induced as a result of stress exposure.

Subsequently, working in the field of psychoneuroendocrinology, Mason and his colleagues contributed toward elucidating the concept of stress and stressors in terms of individual responsivity. The experience of the stress response, within an individual, was viewed not so much as a result of the stimulus itself, but primarily as a result of the perceptions of the individual concerning the stimulus.

The work of Mason and his colleagues also made valuable inroads toward demonstrating the role psychological and emotional factors play in influencing endocrine responses. Since their work, a growing body of data has accumulated which describes the effects of both these factors on the several endocrine components of the body. In fact, it appears that psychological and emotional factors exert an influence on all the endocrine glands and their hormonal secretions. The role that these factors play in the elicitation of the stress response is also well documented. Hence, the data available support the view that stress plays an important role in influencing almost all of the endocrine glands of the body along with the hormones associated with them. In view of the psychological and emotional influences on the endocrine system, the ubiquitous nature of endocrine responses to a wide variety of stressful stimuli assumes crucial importance.

Reports are even available, although scattered, which demonstrate the effects of stress on certain metabolites, nutrients, vitamins, and minerals of the body.

It is important to emphasize that from the brief survey of the research presented in this text, as well as from other scientific investigations, data is available which supports the view that stress can exert its influence at the cellular level (liver cells, various blood cells, etc.) molecular level (glucose in the blood, cholesterol, etc.), tissue level (muscular, coronary, etc.), the organ level (skin, heart, etc.) and the systems level (cardiovascular, immune, gastrointestinal, neuroendocrine, etc.). However, the physiological mechanisms underlying many of the stress induced alterations on various processes of the body awaits continued investigative work.

AFTERWORD

In this text, the attempt has been made to provide an integrative framework from which to survey the complex neuroendocrine mechanisms and psychophysiological processes that comprise what is today called—the stress response.

The pioneer work of Cannon and Selye and the theories of stress and diseases of adaptation which have since emerged, have certainly, in these past years, made significant inroads into the whole field of medical research and practice, to say nothing of their influence in the whole health-care model. This is evidenced by the fact that only a few short years ago, in the 1950s, Selye was the sole author of a treatise on stress. Today there are well over 15,000 research papers and articles written on the subject, and from many different perspectives. The contributions of Cannon, Selye, Mason, and several others, through their studies of individual behavior patterns and psychoneuroendocrine responses, have laid the foundation for a new and emerging science, the science of Stressology.

Back in 1928, Cannon, in addressing his fellow physicians, emphasized the concept that emotional stress, and the means to relieve it, would provide several opportunities for worthwhile studies and research. I believe, in the last 5 decades, we have come a long way in carrying out his suggestion. In the process, many disciplines of science appear to be merging closer together. One witnesses the emergence of a new field of medicine called behavioral medicine, which incorporates several traditional disciplines. Also, an important link in the biomedical and behavioral sciences emphasizes the study of the common pathways by which the central nervous system, the brain, regulates the autonomic nervous system and the endocrine systems. There is much data which supports the roles that these systems play in mediating human responsivity to outside stimuli or various types of stress exposures. Also, the discovery of the neuropeptides in the brain, and their possible interrelationship with endocrine activity in mediating the stress response, provides another new frontier for understanding brain function, endocrine function, and behavior. Perhaps as these different disciplines of biological science merge and are viewed as being more interrelated, the object of their study, the human being, will be seen from a more integrated perspective. Indeed, the once dichotomized mind, body, and spirit may come to be accepted from a much more integrative, holistic, and unified perspective.

REFERENCES

CHAPTER 1

Selye, H. *The physiology and pathology of exposure to stress*. Montreal: Acta Inc., Medical Publishers 1950, 27.

Selye, H. *The stress of life*. London: Longmans, Green, 1957.

Selye, H. *Stress in health and disease*. Reading, Mass: Butterworths, 1976.

CHAPTER 2

Carruthers, M. & Taggart, P. Vagotonicity of violence. *British Medical Journal*, 1973, 3, 384.

Curtis, B.A., Jacobson, S., & Marcus, E.M. *An introduction to neurosciences*. Philadelphia: W.B. Saunders Co., 1972.

Darrow, C.W. Physiological and clinical tests of autonomic functioning and autonomic balance. Physiological Review, 1943, 23, 1.

Engle, G. Sudden and rapid death during psychological stress. *Annals of Internal Medicine* 1971, 74, 771.

Gellhorn, E. Central nervous system tuning and its implications for neuropsychiatry. *Journal of Nervous and Mental Disorders*, 1968, 147, 148.

Guyton, A.C. *Textbook of medical physiology.* Philadelphia: W.B. Saunders, Co., 1981.

MacLean, P.D. Sensory and perceptive factors in emotional functions in the brain. In L. Levi (ed.), *Emotions: Their parameters and measurement.* New York: Raven Press, 1975.

CHAPTER 3

Cannon, W.B. The emergency function of the adrenal medulla in pain and in the major emotion. *American Journal of Physiology* 1914, *33,* 356.

Cannon, W.B., & Paz, D. Emotional stimulation of adrenal gland secretion. *American Journal of Physiology* 1911, *28,* 64.

Duffy E. Activation and behavior. New York: Wiley, 1962.

Henry, J.P., & Stephens, P. *Stress, health and the social environment.* New York. Springer, 1977.

Lacey, J.I. & Lacey, B.C. The relationship of resting autonomic activity to motor impulsivity. *Research Publications of the Association for Nervous and Mental Disease* 1958, *36,* 144(a).

Lacey, J.I., & Lacey, B.C. Verification and extension of the principle of autonomic response — stereotypy. *American Journal of Psychology*, 1958, *71,* 50(b).

Roldan, E., Alvarez-Palaez, P., & de Molina, F. Electrographic study of the amygdaloid defense response. *Physiology and Behavior* 1974, *13,* 779.

Selye, H. The general adaptation syndrome and the gastrointestinal diseases of adaptation. *American Journal of Proctology* 1951, *2,* 167.

Selye, H. *Stress in health and disease. Reading, Mass.: Butterworth's,* 1976.

Wilson, E.S., & Schneider, C. The neurophysiologic pathways of distress. *Stress/Pain Manager Newsletter.* S/P Management Group, Kansas City, Mo., May/June 1981.

CHAPTER 5

Abe, K., Nicholson, W.E., Liddle, G.W., Island, D.P., & Orth, D.N. Radioimmunoassay of beta-MSH in Human Plasma and

Tissues. *Journal of Clinical Investigation*, 1967b, *46*, 1609.

Alexander, D.P., Forsling, M.L., Martin, M.J., Nixon, D.A., Ratcliffe, J.G., Redstone, D., & Turnbridge, D. The effect of maternal hypoxia on fetal pituitary hormone release in the sheep. *Biology of the Neonate,* 1972, *21,* 219.

Alexander, D.P., Britton, H.G., Forsling, M.L., Nixon D.A., & Ratcliffe, J.G. Pituitary and plasma concentrations of adrenocorticotropin, growth hormone, vasopressin and oxytocin in fetal and maternal sheep during the latter half of gestation and the response to hemorrhage. *Biology of the Neonate*, 1974, *24*, 206.

Alexander, D.P., Bashore, R.A., Britton, H.G., & Forsling, M.L. Antidiuretic hormone and oxytocin release and anti-diuretic hormone turnover in the fetus lamb and ewe. *Biology of the Neonate*, 1976, *30*, 80.

Brown, G.M., & Martin, J.B. Corticosterone, prolactin, growth hormone response to handling and new environment in the rat. *Psychosomatic Medicine, 1974, 36*, 241.

Brown, G.M., Schalch, D.S., & Reichlin, S. Patterns of growth hormone and cortisol responses to psychological stress in the squirrel monkey. *Endocrinology*, 1971, *88*, 956.

Chard, T., Hudson, C.N., Edwards, C.R.W., Boyd, N.R.H. Release of oxytocin and vasopressin by the human fetus during labor. *Nature*, 1971, *234*, 352.

Coyne, M.D., & Ekitay, J.I. Effect of ovariectomy on pituitary secretion of ACTH. *Endocrinology* 1969, *85*, 1097.

Czarny, D., James, V.H.T., London, J., & Greenweed, F.C. Corticosteroid and growth hormone response to synthetic lysine vasopressin, natural vasopressin, saline solution, and venopuncture. *Lancet*, 1968, *2*, 126.

Daniel, S.S., Husain, M.R., Millez, J., Stark, R.I., Yeh, M.N., James, L.S., Renal response of fetal lamb to complete occlusion of umbilical cord. *American Journal of Gynecology*, 1978, *131, 514*.

De Vane, G.W., & Porter, J.C. An apparent stress-induced release of arginine vasopressin by human neonates. *Journal of Clinical Endocrinology,* 1980, *51*, 1412.

Guyton, A.C. *Textbook of medical physiology* (6th ed.). Philadelphia: W.B. Saunders Co., 1981.

Gwinup, G., Steinberg, T., King, C.G., & Vernikos-Danellis, J. Vasopressin-induced ACTH secretion in man. *Journal of Clinical Endocrinology & Metabolism*, 1967, *27*, 927.

Henkin, R.I., Knigge, K. Effect of sound on hypothalamic pituitary adrenal axis. *American Journal of Physiology*, 1963, *204*, 710.

Hoppenstein, J.M., Miltenberger, F.W., & Moran, W.H. Jr., The increase in blood levels of vasopressin in infants during birth and surgical procedures. *Surgery, Gynecology & Obstetrics (Chicago)*, 1968, *127*, 966.

Kastin, A.J., Schally, A.V., Viosca, S., & Miller, M.C. MSH Activity in Plasma and Pituitaries of Rats after various Treatments. *Endocrinology*, 1969, *84*, 20.

Kastin, A.J., Arimura, A., Viosca, S., Barrett, L., & Schally, A.V. MSH activity in pituitaries of rats exposed to stress. *Neuroendocrinology*, 1967, *2*, 200.

Kokka, N., Garcia J.F., George, R., & Elliott, H.W. Growth hormone and ACTH secretion: Evidence for an inverse relationship in rats. *Endocrinology*, 1972, *90*, 735.

Kraicer, J. Beraud, G., & Lywood, D.W. Pars Intermedia ACTH and MSH content: Effect of adrenalectomy, gonadectomy, and neurotropic (noise) stress. *Neuroendocrinology 1977*, *23*, 352.

Kraicer, J., Gosbee, J.L., & Bencosme, S.A. Pars intermedia and pars distalis: Two sites of ACTH production in the rat hypophysis. *Neuroendocrinology, 1973*, *11*, 156.

Kraicer, J., & Morris, A.R. In vitro release of ACTH from dispersed rat pars intermedia cells. I. Effect of secretagogues. *Neuroendocrinology*, 197a, *20*, 79.

Kraicer, J., & Morris, A.R. In vitro release of ACTH from dispersed rat pars intermedia cells. II Effect of neurotransmitter substances. *Neuroendocrinology*, 1976b, *21*, 175.

Lenox, F.H., Kant, G.J., Sessions, G.R., Pennington, L.L., Mougey, E.H., & Meyerhoff, J.L. Specific hormonal and neurochemical responses to different stressors. *Neuroendocrinology*, 1980, *30*, 300.

Lerner, A.B. Three Unusual Pigmentary Syndromes. *Archives of Dermatology*, 1961, *3*, 97.

Levi, J., Massry, S.G., & Kleeman, C.R. The requirement of cortisol for the inhibitory effect of norepinephrine on the antidiuretic action of vasopressin. *Proceedings of the Society for Experimental Biology and Medicine*, 1973, *142*, 687.

Mason, J.W., Wool, M.S., Wherry, F.E., Pennington, L.L., Brady, J.V., & Beer, B. Plasma growth hormone response to avoidance sessions in the monkey. *Psychosomatic Medicine*, 1968, *30*, 760.

McCann, S.M., Antunes-Rodrigues, J., Nallar, R., & Valtin, H. Pituitary-Adrenal function in the absence of vasopressin. *Endocrinology*, 1966, *79*, 1058.

Meyer, V., & Knobil, E. Growth hormone secretion in the unanesthetized rhesus monkey in response to noxious stimuli. *Endocrinology*, 1967, *80*, 163.

Miyabo, S., Hisada, T., Asato, T., Mizushima, N., & Ueno, K. Growth hormone and cortisol responses to psychological stress: Comparison of normal and neurotic subjects. *Journal of Clinical Endocrinology and Metabolism,* 1975, *42,* 1158.

Moran, W.H., & Zimmermann, B., Mechanisms of antidiuretic hormone (ADH) control of importance to the surgical patient. *Surgery*, 1967, *62*, 639.

Philbin, D.M., Coggins, C.H., Wilson, N., & Sokoloski, J. Antidiuretic hormone levels during cardiopulmonary bypass. *Journal of Thoracic & Cardiovascular Surgery*, 1977, *73*, 145.

Philbin, D.M., & Coggins, C.H. Plasma antidiuretic hormone levels in cardiac surgical patients during morphine and halothane anesthesia. *Anesthesiology*, 1978, *49*, 95.

Sandman, C.A., Kastin, A.J., Schally, A.V., Kendal, J.W., & Miller, L.H. Neuroendocrine responses to physical and psychological stress. *Journal of Comparative & Physiological Psychology*, 1973, *84*, 386.

Schalach, D.S. The influence of physical stress and exercise on growth hormone and insulin secretion in man. *Journal of Laboratory and Clinical Medicine*, 1967, *69*, 256.

Segar, W.E., & Moore, W.W. The regulation of antidiuretic hormone release in man. Effects of change in position and ambient temperature on blood ADH levels. *Journal of Clinical Investigation*, 1968, *47*, 2143.

Stark, R.I., Daniel, S.S., Husain, R.M., James, L.S., Vade Wiele,

R.L. Arginine Vasopressin during gestation and parturition in sheep fetus. *Biology of the Neonate*, 1979, *35*, 235.

Staub, J.J., Jenkins, J.S., Ratcliffe, J.G., & Landon, J. Comparison of corticotropin and corticosteroid response to lysine vasopressin, insulin, and pyrogen in man. *British Medical Journal*, 1973, *1*, 267.

Sulman, F.G. Chromatophorotropic activity of human blood: review of 1,200 cases. *Journal of Clinical Endocrinology & Metabolism*, 1956, *16*, 755.

Taleisnik, S., & Tomates, M.E. Effect of estrogen on pituitary melanocyte-stimulating hormone content. *Neuroendocrinology*, 1969, *5*, 24.

Thody, A.J., Penny, R.J., Clark, D., & Taylor, C. Development of a radioimmunoassay for alpha-melanocyte-stimulating hormone in the rat. *Journal of Endocrinology*, 1975b, *67*, 385.

Weitzman, R.E., Fisher, D.A., Robillard, J., Erenberg, A., Kennedy, R., & Smith, F. Arginine Vasopressin response to an osmotic stimulus in the fetal sheep. *Pediatric Research*, 1978, *12*, 35.

Wiley, M.K., Pearlmutter, A.F., & Miller, R.E. Decreased adrenal sensitivity to ACTH in the vasopressin-deficient (Brattleboro) rat. *Neuroendocrinology*, 1974, *14*, 257.

CHAPTER 6

Cannon, W.B., & Paz, D. Emotional stimulation of adrenal secretion. *American Journal of Physiology*, 1911, *28*, 64.

Cannon, W.B. The emergency function of the adrenal medulla in pain and in the major emotions. *American Journal of Physiology*, 1914, *33*, 356.

Cannon, W.B. *The wisdom of the body*. New York: W.W. Norton Co., Inc., 1932.

Cardus, D., Vallbona, C., Vogt, F.B., Spencer, W.A., Lipscomb, H.S., & Eik-nes, K.B. Influence of bed-rest on plasma levels of 17-hydroxycorticosteroids. *Aerospace Medicine*, 1965, *36*(6), 524.

Dimsdale, J.E., & Moss, J. Plasma catecholamines in stress and exercise. *Journal of Amerian Medical Association*, 1980, *243*, 340.

Engel, F.L., & Lebovitz, H.E. Extra target organ actions of anterior pituitary hormones. In G.W. Harris, & B.T. Donovan, (Eds.) *The pituitary gland*, (Vol. 2), Berkeley, Calif. University of California Press, 1966, 563.

Frankenhaeuser, M. Experimental approach to the study of catecholamines and emotion. In L. Levi (Ed.), *Emotions, their parameters and measurement*, New York, Raven Press, 1975.

Guyton, A.C. *Textbook of medical physiology*. Philadelphia: W.B. Saunders, Co., 1981.

Katz, F.H. Adrenal function during bed rest. *Aerospace Medicine*, 1964, *35*, 849.

Kolpakov, M.M. In Adaptation to muscular activity and hypokinesia. *Novosibirsk*, 1970, *89*.

Kopin, I., Lake, R., & Ziegler, M. Plasma levels of norepinephrine. *Annals of Internal Medicine*, 1978, *88*, 671.

Kovalenko, E.A., & Popkov, V.L., Kondrat'ev, Y.I., Marlyan, E.S., Galushko, Y.S., Prokhonchukov, A.A., Kazaryan, V.A., Morozova, R.S., Serova, L.V., Potspov, A.V., Romanov, V.S., Pishchik, V.B. Izmenenie funktsii orgainizma pri dlitel' noi gipokinezii. *Patologicheskaia Fiziologiia I Eksperimentalnaia Terapiia (Moskva)*, 1971, *14*(6), 3-9.

Levi, L. Psychosocial stimuli, psychophysiological reactions and disease. *Acta Medica Scandinavia Supplement*, 1972, 528.

Lindsley, D.B. Emotions. In John Wiley, New York: (Ed.), *Handbook of experimental psychology*. 1951.

Mason, J. Emotions as reflected in patterns of endocrine integration. In L. Levi (Ed.), *Emotions, their parameters and measurement, New York: Raven Press, 1975.*

Mason, J.B. *Organization of psychoendocrine mechanisms: A review and reconsideration of research. In N. Greenfield & R. Sternback (Eds.),* Handbook of psychophysiology, New York: Holt, Rinehart & Winston, 1972.

Mason, J.W. A review of psychoendocrine research on the sympathetic-adrenal medullary system. *Psychosomatic Medicine*, 1968a, *30*, 631.

Mason, J.W. Organization of psychoendocrine mechanisms. *Psychosomatic Medicine*, 1968b, *30*.

Mason, J.W. A review of psychoendocrine research on the pituitary adrenal cortical system. *Psychsomatic Medicine*, 1968c, *30*, 576.

Mason, J.W., Mahler, J.T., Hartley, L.H., Maugey, E.M., Perlow' M.J., & Jones, L.G. Selectivity of corticosteroid and catecholamine response to various natural stimuli. In G. Serban (Ed.), *Psychopathology of human adaptation*, New York: Plenum Press, 1976.

Roessler, R., & Greenfield, M. (Eds.). *Physiological correlates of psychological disorders*, Madison, Wis.: University of Wisconsin Press, 1962.

Selye, H. Stress. The physiology and pathology of exposure to stress. Montreal: *Acta Inc.*, Medical Publishers, 1950.

Selye, H. The general adaptation syndrome and the gastrointestinal diseases of adaptation, *American Journal of Proctology*, 1951, *2*, 167.

Selye, H. *The stress of life*. New York: McGraw-Hill, 1956.

Selye, H. *Stress in health and disease*. Reading, Mass:, Butterworths, 1976.

Tavadyan, D.S., & Goncharov, N.P., Dynamics of blood levels of aldosterone and of cortisol and its precursors in Macaca rhesus during prolongedhypokinesia. *Eksperimental 'noi Biologii i Meditieny*, 1980, *90*, 663.

Wenger, M.A., Clemens, T., Darsie, M.C., Engel, B.T., Estess, F.M. & Sonnenschein, R.R. Autonomic response patterns during intravenous infusion of epinephrine and norepinephrine. *Psychosomatic Medicine*, 1960, *22*, 294.

CHAPTER 7

Bansi, H.W., Kracht, J., Kracht, U., & Meissner, J. Zur Entstehung des Morbus Basedow. *Deutsche Medizinische Wochenschrift*, 1953, *78*, 256.

Blount, H.D., & Hardy, J.D. Thyroid function and surgical trauma as evaluated by iodine conversion ratio. *American Journal of Medical Science*, 1952, *224*, 112.

Bogoroch, R., & Timiras, P. The response of the thyroid gland of the rat to severe stress. *Endocrinology*, 1951, *49*, 548.

Brown, M.R., & Hedge, G.A. Multiple effects of glucocorticoids on TSH secretion in unaesthetized rats. *Endocrinology*, 1973, *92*, 1305.

Brown-Grant, K., & Pethes, G. Stress and the guinea-pig thyroid. *Journal of Physiology*, (London), 1960, *151*, 40.

Burr, W.A., Griffiths, R.S., Black, E.G., & Hoffenberg, R. Serum triiodothyronine and reverse triiodothyronine concentrations after surgical operation. *Lancet*, 1975, *2*, 1277.

Chan, V., Wang, C., & Yeung, T.T.T. Pituitary-Thyroid responses to surgical stress. *Acta Endocrinologia*, 1978, *88*, 490.

Charters, A.C., Odell, W.D., & Thompson, J.C. Anterior pituitary function during surgical stress and convalescence. Radioimmunoassay measurement of blood TSH, LH, FSH and growth hormone. *Journal of Clinical Endocrinology and Metabolism*, 1969, *29*, 63.

D'Angelo, S.A. Adenohypophyseal function in the guinea pig at low environmental temperature. *Federation Proceedings*, 1960a, *19*, 51.

D'Angelo, S.A. Hypothalamus and endocrine function in persistent estrous rats at low environmental temperature. *American Journal of Physiology*, 1960b, *199*, 701.

Dewhurst, K.E., El Kabir, D.J., Harris, G.W., & Mandelbrote, B.M. A review of the effect of stress on the activity of the central nervous-pituitary-thyroid axis in animals and man. *Confinia Neurologica*, 1968, *30*, 161.

Döhler, K.D., Gartner, K., von zur Muhler, A., & Dohler, U. Activation of anterior pituitary thyroid and adrenal gland in rats after disturbance stress. *Acta Endocrinologia*, 1977, *86*, 486.

Ducommun, P., Vale, W., Sakiz, E., & Guillemin, R. Reversal of the inhibition of TSH secretion due to acute stress. *Endocrinology*, 1967, *80*, 953.

Eickhoff, W. Über den experimentellen nervosen Vollbasedow. *Zentralblatt fuer Allgemeine Patholigic und Pathologische Anatomie*, 1949, *85*, 112.

Eickhoff, W. Über den experimentellen nervosen Vollbasedow. *Ver handlungen Der Deutschen & Gesellschaft Fur Pathologie.*, 1950, *32*, 295.

Engstrom, W.W., & Markardt, B. *Journal of Clinical Investigation*, 1954, *33*, 931.

Goldenberg, I.S., Hayes, M.A., & Greene, N.M. Endocrine responses during operative procedures. *Annals of Surgery*, 1959, *150*, 196.

Goldenberg, I.S., Lutwak, L., Rosenbaum, P.J., & Hayes, M.A. Thyroid-adrenocortical inter-relations following operation. *Surgery, Gynecology and Obstetrics*, 1954, *98*, 513.

Goldenberg, I.S., Lutwak, L., Rosenbaum, P.J., & Hayes, M.A. Thyroid-adrenocortical metabolic inter-relations. *Journal of Clinical Endocrinology*, 1955, *15*, 227.

Goldenberg, I.S., Rosenbaum, P.J., Lutwak, L., & Hayes, M.A. Thyroid activity during operation. *Surgery, Gynecology & Obstetrics*, 1956, *102*, 128.

Goldenberg, I.S., Rosenbaum, P.J., White, C., & Hayes, M.A. The effect of operative trauma on the utilization of thyroid hormone. *Surgery, Gynecology & Obstetrics*, 1957, *104, 295*.

Greene, N.M., & Goldenberg, I.S. The effect of anesthesia on thyroid activity in humans. Anesthesiology, 1959, 20, 125.

Harland, W.A., Horton, P.W., Strang, R., Fitzgerald, B., Richards, J.R., & Holloway, K.B. Release of thyroxine from the liver during anesthesia and surgery. *British Journal of Anaesthesiology*, 1974, *46*, 818.

Kirby, R., Clark, F., & Johnston, I.D.A. The effect of surgical operation of moderate severity on thyroid function. *Clinical Endocrinology*, 1973, *2*, 89.

Langer, P., & Lichardus, B. Thyroid function and its fluctuations during and after short-term stress and dexamethasone administration in rats. *Neuroendocrinology*, 1969, *4*, 112.

Mason, J.W., Brady, J.V., Tolson, W.W., Robinson, J.A., Taylor, E.D., & Mougey, E.H. Patterns of thyroid gonadal and adrenal hormone secretion related to psychological stress in the monkey. *Psychosomatic Medicine*, 1961, *23*, 446.

Oyama, T., Shibata, S., & Matsuki, A. Thyroxine distribution during ether and thiopental anesthesia in man. *Anesthesia & Analgesia*, 1969, *48*, 1.

Oyama, T., Taniguchi, K., Ishihara, H., Matsuki, A., Maeda, A., Murakawa, T., & Kudo, T. Effects of enflurane anesthesia and surgery on endocrine function in man. *British Journal of Anesthesiology*, 1979, *51*, 141.

Perry, W.F., & Gemmell, J.P. The effect of surgical operations on the excretion of iodine, corticosteroids and uric acid. *Canadian Journal of Research*, 1949, *27*, 320.

Pollard, I., Bassett, J.R., & Cairncross, K.D. Plasma thyroid hormone and glucocorticoid concentration on the male rat following prolonged exposure to stress. *Australian Journal of Biological Science, 1979, 32*, 237.

Ramsden, D.B., Smith, T.J., Burr, W.A., Black, E.G., Lee, J.M., & Hoffenberg, R. Effects of surgical stress and corticotropin on the peripheral metabolism of thyroid hormones in rabbits. *Journal of Endocrinology*, 1979, *82*, 403.

Reichlin, S., & Glaser, R.I. Thyroid function in experimental streptococcal pneumonia in the rat. *Journal of Experimental Medicine*, 1958, *107*, 219.

Reichlin, S. & Control of thyrotropic secretion. In Martini, L. & Ganong, W.F. (Eds.). *Neuroendocrinology*. London: Academic Press, 1966.

Sakiz, E., & Guillemin, R. Inverse effects of purified hypothalamic TRF on the acute secretion of TSH and ACTH. *Endocrinology*, 1965, *77*, 797.

Schwartz, A.E., & Roberts, K.E. Alternations in thyroid function following surgical trauma. *Surgery*, 1957, *42*, 814.

Shambaugh, G.E., & Beisel, W.R. Alterations in thyroid physiology during pneumococcal septicemia in the rat. *Endocrinology*, 1966, *79*, 511.

Sternberg, T.H., Newcomer, V.D., Steffen, C.G., Fields, M., & Libby, R.L. Distribution of radioactive iodine (131) in experimental coccidioidomycoses and sporotrichosis. *Journal of Investigative Dermatology*, 1955, *24*, 397.

Surks, M.I., & Oppenheimer, J.H. Postoperative changes in the concentration of thyroxine-binding prealbumin and serum-free thyroxine. *Journal of Endocrinology*, 1964, *24*, 794.

Van Middlesworth, C., & Berry, M.M. Iodine metabolism during anoxia, nephrectomy, trauma, avitaminoses and starvation in the rat. *American Journal of Physiology*, 1951, *167*, 576.

Williams, R.H., Jaffe, H., & Kemp, C. Effect of severe stress upon thyroid function. *American Journal of Physiology*, 1949, *159*, 291.

CHAPTER 8

Cheah, K.S., & Cheah, A.M., The trigger for PSE condition in stress-susceptible pigs. *Journal of the Science of Food and Agriculture*, 1976, *27*, 1137.

Cheah, K.S., & Cheah, A.M. Mitochondrial calcium efflux and porcine stress-susceptibility. *Experientia*, 1979, *35*, 1001.

Hofman, P., Schwille, P.O., & Thun, R. Hypocalcemia during restraint stress in rats. *Research in Experimental Medicine*, 1979, *175*, 159.

Schwille, P.O., Schellerer, W., Reitzenstein, M., & Hermanek, P. Hyperglucagonemia, hypocalcemia and diminished gastric mucosal blood flow-evidence for an etiological role in stress ulcer formation of rat. *Experientia*, 1974, *30*, 824.

Schwille, P.O., & Putz, F.J., Thun, R., Schellerer, W., Draxler, G., & Lang, G. Anti-stress ulcer and anti-secretory effect of somatostatin in rats—failure to suppress endogenous serum gastrin. *Acta Hepato-Gastroenterology*, 1977, *24*, 259.

Schwille, P.O., Steiner, H., Samberger, N.M., & Schellerer, W. Role of calcitonin in stress ulcer formation of various rat models. Preliminary report. *Research in Experimental Medicine*, 1975, *165*, 291.

Tigranian, R.A., Orloff, L.L. Kalita, L.F., Davydova, N.A., & Pavlova, E.A. Changes of blood levels of several hormones, catecholamines, prostaglandins, electrolytes and cAMP in man during emotional stress. *Endocrinologia Experimentialis*, 1980, *14*, 101.

CHAPTER 9

Abplanalp, J.M., Livingston, L., Rose, R.M., & Sandwisch, D. Cortisol and growth hormone responses to psychological stress during the menstrual cycle. *Psychosomatic Medicine*, 1977, *39*, 158.

Ajika, K., Kalra, S.P., Fawcett, C.P., Krulich, L., & McCann, S.M. The effect of stress and nembutal on plasma levels of gonadotropins and prolactin in ovariectomized rats. *Endocrinology*, 1972, *90*, 707.

Andrews, R.V. Effects of climate and social pressure on the adrenal response of lemmings, voles, and mice. *Acta Endocrinologica* (Kbh), 1970, *65, 639.*

Aono, T., Kurachi, K., Miyata, M., Nakashima, A., Koshiyama, K., Uozumi, T., Matusmo, K. Influence of surgical stress under general anesthesia on serum gonadotropin levels in male and female appepatients. *Journal of Clinical Endocrinology and Metabolism,* 1976, *42,* 144.

Aubert, M.L., Lemarchand-Beraud, T., Deguillaume, R., & Desaulles. Cortisol secretion during the normal menstrual cycle. *Acta Endocrinologica,* Copenhagen, 1971, *155,* 78.

Bardin, C.W., & Peterson, R.E. Studies of androgen production by the rat: testosterone and rostenedione content of blood. *Endocrinology,* 1967, *80,* 38.

Bliss, E.L., Frischat, A., & Samuels, I. Brain and Testicular Function. *Life Science,* 1972, *2,* 231.

Blizard, D.A., Slater, J., Liang, B. & Shenkman, L. Serum prolactin and hypothalamic dopamine in rat strains selectively bred for differences in susceptibility to stress. *Neuroendocrinology,* 1977, *23,* 297.

Brown, B., Dettmar, P.W., Dobson, P.R., Lynn, A.G., Metcalf, G., & Morgan, B.A. Opiate analgesics: the effect of agonist-antagonist character on prolactin secretion. *Journal of Pharmacy & Pharmacology,* 1978, *30,* 644.

Carstensen, H., Amer, I., Wide, I., & Amer, B. Plasma testosterone, LH and FSH during the first 24 hours after surgical operations. *Journal of Steroid Biochemistry,* 1973, *4,* 605.

Catt, K.J., Tsuruhara, T., Mendelson, C., Ketelslegers, J.M., & Dufau, M.L. Gonadotropin binding and activation of the interstitial cells of testis. In M.L. Dufau & A.R. Means (Eds.). *Hormone binding and target cell activation in the testis.* New York: Plasma Press, 1976.

Charters, A.C., Odell, W.D., & Thompson, J.C. Anterior pituitary function during surgical stress and convalescence, radioimmunoassay measurement of blood TSH, LH, FSH, and growth hormone. *Journal of Endocrinology,* 1969, *29,* 63.

Chen, C.L., & Meites, J. Effects of estrogen and progesterone on serum and pituitary prolactin levels in ovariectomized rats. *Endocrinology*, 1970, *86*, 503.

Christian, J.J. Population density and reproduction efficiency. *Biology of Reproduction* 1971, *4*, 248.

Conti, C., Sorcini, G., Sciarra, F., Concolino, G., & Lotti, P. Plasma testosterone levels in normal subjects and in hirsute women during adrenal and gonadal function tests. *Research on steroids*: the transaction of the International Symposium on Steroids, 1963.

Dahlöff, L., Hard, E., & Larsson, K. Influence of maternal stress on the development of the fetal genital system. *Physiology and Behavior*, 1978, *20*, 193.

Davidson, J.M., Smith, E., & Levine, S. Testosterone. In H. Ursin, E. Baade, & A. Levine, (Eds.), *Psychology of stress: A study of coping men*. New York: Academic Press, 1978.

de Loos, W.S., Bohus, B., de Jong, W., & de Wied, D. Reduction of heart-rate reactions to emotional stress by ovarian hormones in rats. Proceedings of the Society for Endocrinology, Abstract 138P, 1979.

Du Ruisseau, P., Taché, Y., Selye, H., Ducharme, J.R., & Collu, R. Effects of chronic stress on pituitary hormone release induced by combined hemi-extirpation of the thyroid, adrenal and ovary in rats. *Neuroendocrinology*, 1977, *24*, 169.

Du Ruisseau, P., Taché, Y., Brazeau, P., & Collu, R. Pattern of adrenohypophyseal hormone change induced by various stressors in female and male rats. *Neuroendocrinology*, 1978, *27*, 257.

Ellis, B.W., Evans, P.F., Phillips, P.D., Murray, M.A.F., Jacobs, H.S., James, V.H.T., & Dudley, H.A.F. Effects of surgery on plasma testosterone, luteinizing hormone and follicle-stimulating hormone: a comparison of pre- and postoperative patterns of secretions. *Journal of Endocrinology*, 1976, *69*, 25A.

Euker, J.S., Meites, J., & Reigle, G.D. Effect of acute stress on serum LH and prolactin in intact, castrated and dexamethasone-treated rats. *Endocrinology*, 1975, *96*, 85.

Ferland, L., Kledzik, G.S., Cusan, L., & Labrie, F. Evidence for a role of endorphins in stress- and suckling-induced prolactin release in the Rat. *Molecular and Cellular Endocrinology*, 1978, *12*, 267.

Frantz, A.G., Kleinberg, D.L., & Noel, G.L. Studies on prolactin in man. *Recent Progress in Hormone Research*, 1972, *28*, 527.

Genazzani, A.R., Lemarchand-Beraud, T. Aubert, M.L., & Felber, J.P. Pattern of ACTH, hGH and cortisol during menstrual cycle. *Journal of Clinical Endocrinology & Metabolism*, 1975, *49*, 431.

Gray, G.D., Smith, E.R., Damassa, D.A., Ehrenkrantz, J.R.L., & Davidson, J.M. Neuroendocrine mechanisms mediating the suppression of circulating testosterone levels associated with chronic stress in male rats. *Neuroendocrinology*, 1978, *25*, 247.

Guyton, A.C. *Textbook of Medical Physiology*, (6th ed.). Philadelphia: W. B. Saunders Co., 1981.

Jobin, M., Feland, L., Cote, J., & Labrie, R. Effect of exposure to cold on hypothalamic TRH and plasma levels of TSH and prolactin in the rat. *Neuroendocrinology, 1975, 18*, 204.

Kalra, P.S., Fawcett, C.P., Krulich, L., & McCann, S.M. The effects of gonadal steroids on plasma gonadotropins and prolactin in the rat. *Endocrinology*, 1973, *92*, 1256.

Koenig, J.I., Mayfield, M.A., McCann, S.M., & Krulich, L. Stimulation of prolactin secretion by morphine: role of the central serotonergic system. *Life Sciences*, 1979, *25*, 853.

Koninckx, P. Stress hyperprolactianemia in clinical practice. *Lancet* 1978, *1*, 273.

Kreuz, L.E., Rose, R.M., & Jennings, J.R. Suppression of plasma testosterone levels and psychological stress. *Archives of General Psychiatry*, 1972, *26*, 479.

Krulich, L., Hefco, E., Illner, P., & Read, C.B. The effects of acute stress on the secretion of LH, FSH, Prolactin and GH in the normal male rat with comments on their statistical evaluation. *Neuroendocrinology*, 1974, *16*, 293.

Lisk, R.D. Progesterone — role in limitation of ovulation and sex behavior in mammals. *Transactions of the New York Academy of Science*, 1969, *39*, 593.

Lu, K.H., Shaar, C.J., Kortright, K.H., & Meites, J. Effects of synthetic TRH on in vitro and in vivo prolactin release in the rat. *Endocrinology*, 1972, *91*, 1540.

Marinari, K.T., Leshner, A.I., & Doyle, M.P. Menstrual cycle status and adrenocortical reactivity to psychological stress. *Psychoneuroendocrinology*, 1976, *1*, 213.

Martin, J.B., Tolis, G., Woods, I., & Guyda, H. Failure of naloxone to influence physiological growth hormone and prolactin secretion. *Brain Research*, 1979, *168*, 210.

Matsumoto, K., Takeyasu, K., Mizutani, S., Hamanaka, Y., & Uozumi, T. Plasma testosterone levels following surgical stress in male patients. *Acta Endocrinologica*, 1970, *65*, 11.

Meites, J., Nicoll, C.S. & Talwalker, P.K. *Advances in Neuroendocrinology*, 238. Urbana, IL: University of Illinois Press, 1963.

Meltzer, H.Y., Miller, R.J., Fessler, R.G., Simonovic, M., & Fang, V.S. Effects of enkephalin in analogues on prolactin release in the rat. *Life Sciences*, 1978, *22*, 1931.

Monden, Y., Koshiyama, K., Tanaka, H., Mizutani, S., Aono, T., Hamanaka, Y., Uozumi, T., & Matsumoto, K. Influence of major surgical stress on plasma testosterone, plasma LH and urinary steroids. *Acta Endocrinologica*, 1972, *69*, 542.

Nakashima, A., Koshiyama, K., Uozumi, T., Monden, T., Hamanaka, Y., Kurachi, K., Aono, T., Mizutani, S., & Matsumoto, K. Effects of general anesthesia and severity of surgical stress on serum LH and testosterone in males. *Acta Endocrinologica*, 1975, *78*, 258.

Neill, J.D. Effect of "stress' on serum prolactin and luteinizing hormone levels during the estrous cycle of the rat. *Endocrinology*, 1970, *87*, 1192.

Nequin, L.G., & Schwartz, N.B. Adrenal participation in the timing of mating and LH release in the cyclic rat. *Endocrinology*, 1971, *88*, 325.

Noel, G.L., Suh, H.K., Stone, G., & Frantz, A.G. Human prolactin and growth hormone release during surgery and other conditions of stress. *Journal of Clinical Endocrinology and Metabolism*, 1972, *35*, 840.

Noel, G.L., Dimond, R.C., Earll, J.M., & Frantz, A.G. Prolactin,

Thyrotropin, and Growth Hormone release during stress associated with parachute jumping. *Aviation, Space and Environmental Medicine*, 1976, *47*, 543.

Peyser, M.R., Ayalon, D., Harell, A., Toof, R., & Cordova, T. Stress induced delay of ovulation. *Obstetrics & Gynecology*, 1973, *42*, 667.

Piercy, M., & Shin, S.H. Comparative studies of prolactin secretion in estradiol-primed and normal male rats induced by ether stress, pimozide and TRH. *Neuroendocrinology*, 1980, *31*, 270.

Ragavan, V.V. & Frantz, A.G. Suppression of serum prolactin by naloxone but not by anti-β-Endorphin antiserum in stressed and unstressed rats. *Life Sciences*, 1981, *28*, 921.

Ratner, A., Talwalker, P.K., & Meites, J. Effect of estrogen administration in vivo and prolactin release by rat pituitary in vitro. *Proceedings of the Society for Experimental Biology & Medicine*, 1963, *112*, 12.

Repcekova D., & Milulaj, L. Plasma testosterone of rats subjected to immobilization stress and/or HCG administration. *Hormone Research*, 1977, *8*, 51.

Riegle, G.D., & Meites, J. The effect of stress on serum prolactin in the female rat. *Proceedings of the Society for Experimental Biology & Medicine*, 1976, *152*, 441.

Rivier, C., Vale, W., Ling, N., Brown, M., & Guillemin, R. Stimulation in vivo of the secretion of prolactin and growth hormone by beta-endorphin. *Endocrinology*, 1977, *100*, 238.

Rose, R.M., Gordon, T.P., & Bernstein, I.S. Plasma testosterone levels in the male rhesus monkey: influence of sexual and social stimuli; *Science*, 1972, *178*, 643.

Rossier, J., French, E., Rivier, C., Shibasaki, T., Guillemin, R., & Bloom, F.E. Stress-induced release of prolactin: blockade by dexamethasone and naloxone may indicate β-endorphin mediation. *Proceedings of the National Academy of Science, USA*, 1980, 77, 666.

Saez, J.M., Morera, A.M., Haour, F., & Evain, D. Effects of in vivo administration of dexamethasone, corticotropin and human chorionic gonadotropin on testicular interstitial cells in prepubertal rats. *Endocrinology*, 1977, *101*, 1256.

Saxena, B.N., Dusitsin, N., & Lazarus, L. Human growth hormone, thyroid stimulating hormone and cortisol levels in the serum of menstruating Thai women. *Journal of Obstetrics & Gynecology of the British Commonwealth*, 1974, *81*, 563.

Selye, H. *Stress in health and disease*, Butterworths, Reading, Mass., 1976.

Shaar, C.J., Frederickson, R.C., Dininger, N.B., & Jackson, L. Enkephalin analogues and naloxone modulate the release of growth hormone and prolactin — evidence for regulation by an endogenous opioid peptide in the brain. *Life Sciences*, 1977, *21*, 853.

Shin, S.H. Thyrotropin releasing hormone (TRH) is not the physiological prolactin releasing factor (PRF) in the male rat. *Life Sciences*, 1978, *23*, 1813.

Shin, S.H. Prolactin secretion in acute stress is controlled by prolactin releasing factor. *Life Sciences*, 1979, *25*, 1829.

Shin, S.H. Estradiol generates pulses of prolactin secretion in castrated male rats. *Neuroendocrinology*, 1979, *29*, 270.

Sorcini, G., Sciarra, F., Concolino, G., & Rascio, L. Effect of ACTH on plasma testosterone in normal human subjects. *Folia Endocrinologica*, 1963, *16*, 449.

Sorcini, G., Fraioli, F., Panunzi, C., Rotolo, A., & Sciarra, F. Surgical stress: decrease in plasma testosterone levels due to hypersecretion of ACTH? *Folia Endocrinologica*, Roma, 1974, *27*, (6pt2), 685.

Stevens, R.W., & Lawson, D.M. The influence of estrogen on plasma prolactin levels induced by thyrotropin releasing hormone (TRH), clonidine and serotonin in ovariectomized rats. *Life Sciences*, 1977, *20*, 216.

Taché, Y., Du Ruisseau, P., Selye, H., Taché, J., & Collu, R. Shift in adrenohypophyseal activity during chronic intermittent immobilization of rats. *Neuroendocrinology*, 1976, *22*, 325.

Taché, Y., Du Ruisseau, P., Ducharme, J.R., & Collu, R. Pattern of adrenohypophyseal hormone changes in male rats following chronic stress. *Neuroendocrinology*, 1978, *26*, 208.

Taché, Y. Du Ruisseau, P. Ducharme, J.R. & Collu, R. Adrenohypophyseal hormone response to chronic stress in dexamethasone-treated rats, *Hormone Research*, 1979, *11*, 101.

Taché, Y., Durcharme, J.R. Charpenet, G., Haour, F., Saez, J., & Collu, R. Effects of chronic intermittent immobilization stress on hypophyso-gonadal function of rats. *Acta Endocrinologica*, 1980, *93*, 168.

Tanaka, H., Manabe, H., Koshiyama, K., Hamanaka, Y., Matsumoto, K., & Uozumi, T. Excretion patterns of 17-ketosteroids and 17-hydroxycorticosteroids in surgical stress. *Acta Endocrinologica*, 1970, *65*, 1.

Tashjian, A.M., Barowsky, N.F., & Jensen, D.K. Direct evidence for stimulation of prolactin by pituitary cells in culture. *Biochemical & Biophysical Research Communications*, 1971, *43*, 516.

Thomas, T.R., & Gerall, A.A. Dissociation of reproductive physiology and behavior induced by neonatal treatment with steroids. *Endocrinology*, 1969, *85*, 781.

Tigranian, R.A., Orloff, L.L., Kalita, N.F., Davydova, N.A., & Pavlova, E.A. Changes of blood levels of several hormones, catecholamines, prostaglandins, electrolytes and cAMP in man during emotional stress, *Endocrinologia Experimentalis*, 1980, *14*, 101.

Tolis, G. Hickey, J., & Guyda, H. Effects of morphine on serum growth hormone, cortisol, prolactin and thyroid stimulating hormone in man. *Journal of Clinical Endocrinology & Metabolism*, 1975, *41*, 797.

Turpen, C., Johnson, D.C., & Dunn, J.D. Stress-induced gonadotropin and prolactin secretory patterns. *Neuroendocrinology*, 1976, *20*, 339.

Valverde-R., C., Chieffo, V., & Reichlin, S. Failure of response to block ether-induced release of prolactin: physiological evidence that stress induced prolactin release is not caused by acute inhibition of PIF secretion. *Life Sciences*, 1973, *12*, 327.

Van Vugt, D.A., Bruni, J.F., & Meites, J. Nalaxone inhibition of stress-induced increase in prolactin secretion. *Life Sciences*, 1978, *22*, 85.

von Eiff, A.W., Plotz, E.J., Beck, K.J., & Czernik, A. The effect of estrogens and progestins on blood pressure regulation of normotensive women. *American Journal of Obstetrics & Gynecology*, 1971, *109*, 887.

von Eiff, A.W., & Piekarski, C. Stress reactions of normotensives and hypertensives and the influence of female sex hormones on blood pressure regulation. *Progress in Brain Research*, 1977, *47*, 289.

CHAPTER 10

Allison, S.P., Tomlin, P.F., & Camberlain, M.J. Some effects of anesthesia and surgery on carbohydrate and fat metabolism. *British Journal of Anaesthesiology*, 1969, *41*, 588.

Ashby, M.M., Heath, D.F., & Stoner, H.G. A quantitative study of carbohydrate metabolism in the normal and injured rat. *Journal of Physiology*, London, 1965, *179*, 193.

Bloom, S.R., Daniel, P.M., Johnston, D.I., Ogawa, O., & Pratt, O.E. Release of glucagon induced by stress. *Quarterly Journal of Experimental Physiology*, 1973, *58*, 99.

Brockman, R.P., & Bergman, E.N. Effect of glucagon on plasma alanine and glutamine metabolism and hepatic gluconeogenesis in sheep. *American Journal of Physiology*, 1975, *228*, 1627.

Brockman, R.P. & Manns, J.G. Effect of trauma on plasma glucagon and insulin concentrations in sheep. *Canadian Journal of Comparative Medicine*, 1976, *40*, 5.

Clarke, R.S.J. The hyperglycemic response to different types of surgery and anesthesia. *British Journal of Anaesthesiology*, 1970, *42*, 45.

Giddings, A.E.B., Mangnall, D., Rowland, B.J., & Clark, R.G. Plasma insulin and surgery. 1. Early changes due to operation in the insulin response to glucose. *Annals of Surgery*, 1977, *186*, 681.

Halter, J.B., Pflug, A.E., & Porte, Jr., D. Mechanism of plasma catecholamine increases during surgical stress in man. *Journal of Clinical Endocrinology & Metabolism*, 1977, *45*, 936.

Halter, J.B., & Pflug, A.E. Relationship of impaired insulin secretion during surgical stress to anesthesia and catecholamine release. *Journal of Clinical Endocrinology & Metabolism*, 1980, *51*, 1093.

Ichikawa, Y., Kawagoe, M., Nishikai, M., Yoskida, K., & Homma, M. Plasma corticotropin (ACTH), growth hormone (GH), and 11-OHCS (hydroxycorticosteroid) response during surgery. *Journal of Laboratory & Clinical Medicine*, 1971, *78*, 882.

Madsen, S.N., Fog-Moller, F., Christiansen, C., Vester-Ander-
son, T., & Enquist, A. Cyclic AMP, adrenaline and noradrenaline in plasma during surgery. *British Journal of Surgery*,
1978, *65*, 191.

Newsome, H.H., & Rose, J.C. The response of human adrenocorticotropic hormone and growth hormone to surgical stress, *Journal of Clinical Endocrinology & Metabolism*, 1971, *33*, 481.

Nijjar, M.S., & Perry, W.F. Effect of trauma on serum insulin
levels in rabbits. *Diabetologica*, 1971, 7, 357.

Noel, G.L., Suh, H.K., Stone, J.G., & Frantz, A.G. Human prolactin and growth hormone release during surgery and other
conditions of stress. *Journal of Clinical Endocrinology &
Metabolism*, 1972, *35*, 840.

Phillips, R.W., House, W.A., Miller, R.A., Mott, J.L., & Sooby,
D.L. Fatty acid, epinephrine and glucagon hyperglycemia in
normal and depancreatized sheep. *American Journal of Physiology*,
1969, *217*, 1265.

West, C.E., & Passey, R.F. Effect of glucose load and of insulin on
the metabolism of glucose and of palmitate in sheep. *Biochemical
Journal*, 1967, *102*, 58.

Yamaguchi, K., & Matsuoka, A. Effects of a high fat diet and
electric stress on adenylate cyclase activity and insulin release in
isolated islets of Langerhans. *Hormone & Metabolic Research*, 1982,
14, 117.

CHAPTER 11

Bindoni, M., Jutisz, M., & Ribot, C. Characterization and partial
purification of a substance in the pineal gland which inhibits cell
multiplication in vitro. *Biochimica et Biophysica Acta*, 1976, *437*,
577.

Bostelmann, W., Gocke, H., Ernst, B., & Tesmann, D. Der Eif-
lubeiner Melatoninbehandlung auf das Wachstum des Walker
Carcinosarcoma der Ratte. *Zentralblatt fuer Allgemeine Pathologie
und Pathologische Anatomie*, 1971, *114*, 289.

Brodan, V., Kuhn, E., Veselková, A., & Kaucká, J. The effect of
stress on circadian rhythms. *Czechoslovak Medicine*, 1982, *1*, 1.

Buswell, R.S. The pineal and neoplasia. *Lancet*, 1975, I: *34*.

De Marzo, V., Panizarri, G.P., & Vegeto, A. Crescità tumorale e ormone epifisario. Studio sperimentale. *Archivio Italiano Di Patologia E Clinica Dei Tumori*, 1958, *2*, 1308.

Dunn, J.D. Circadian variation in adrenocortical and anterior pituitary hormones. In M. Kawakami (Ed.). *Biological rhythms in neuroendocrine activity*, Tokyo: Igaku Shoin, 1974.

Halberg, F., Halberg, E., Barnum, C.P. & Bittner, J.J. Physiologic 24-hour periodicity in human beings and mice, the lighting regimen, and daily routine. Photoperiodism and related phenomena in plants and animals. Washington, D.C., *American Association for the Advancement of Science Publication*, 1959, *55*, 803.

Halberg, F. Chronobiology. *Annals of Physiology*, 1969, *31*, 675.

Huxley, M., & Tapp, E. Effects of biogenic amines on the growth of rat tumors. *Life Science*, 1972, *11*, 19.

Kanabrocki, E.L., Scheving, L.E., Halberg, F., Brewer, R.L., & Bird, R.J. Circadian variations in presumably healthy young soldiers. National Technical Information Service, US Department of Commerce, Document PB 228427, 1974.

Krieger, D.T. Effect of neonatal hydrocortisone on corticosteroid circadian periodicity, responsivness to ACTH and stress on prepuberal and adult rats. *Neuroendocrinolgy*, 1974, *16*, 355.

Krieger, D.T. Circadian pituitary adrenal rhythms. Biological rhythms and endocrine function. Hedlund, L.W.; Franz, J.M.; and Kenny, A.D. (Eds.) *Advances in Experimental Medicine & Biology*, 1975, *54*, 169.

Kvetnansky, R., Kopin, I.J., & Klein, D.C. Stress increases pineal epinephrine. *Communications in Psychopharmacology*, 1979, *3*, 69.

Lapin, V. Pineal gland and malignancy. *Oesterreichische Zeitschrift Fur Onkologie*, 1976, *3*, 51.

Lynch, H.J., Eng, J.P., & Wurtman, R.J. Control of pineal indole biosynthesis by changes in sympathetic tone caused by factors other than environmental lighting. *Proceedings of the National Academy of Sciences*, 1973a, *70*, 1704.

Lynch, H.J., Ho, M., & Wurtman, R.J. The adrenal medulla may mediate the increase in pineal melatonin synthesis induced stress but not that caused by exposure to darkness. *Journal of Neural Transmission*, 1977, *40*, 87.

Lynch, H.J., Jimerson, D.C., Ozaki, Y., Post, R.M., Bunney,

W.E., Jr., & Wurtman, R.J. Entertainment of rhythmic melatonin secretion in man to a 12-hour phase shift in the light/dark
cycle. *Life Sciences*, 1978, *23*, 1557.

Miline, R. The role of the pineal gland in stress. *Journal of Neural
Transmission*, 1980, *47*, 191.

Quay, W.B., & Gorray, K.C. Pineal effects on metabolism and
glucose homeostasis: evidence for lines of humoral mediation of
pineal influences on tumor growth. *Journal of Neural Transmission*, 1980, *47*, 107.

Selye, H. *The physiology and pathology of exposure to stress*, Montreal:
Acta Inc., Medical Publishers, 1950.

Sollberger, A. *A biological rhythm research*. Amsterdam, London,
New York: Elsevier Publishing Co. 1965.

Steinbach, G., Hilfenhaus, M., Mayersbach, H.v., & Poesche, W.
Circadian influences on clinical values in man. *Archives of Tox-
icology*, 1976, *36*, 317.

Steinman, A.M., Smerin, S.E., & Barchas, J.D. Epinephrine
metabolism in mammalian brain after intravenous and intraven-
tricular administration. *Science*, 1969, *165*, 616.

Taylor, A.N., Lorenz, R.J., Turner, B.B., Ronnekleiv, O.K.,
Casady, R.L., & Branch, B.J. Factors influencing pituitary-
adrenal rhythmicity: its ontogeny and circadian variations in
stress responsiveness. *Psychoneuroendocrinology*, 1976, *1*, 291.

Vaughan, G.M., Allen, J.P., Tullis, W., Sackman, J.W., & Vaughan, M.K. Stress-induced increase of pineal acetyltransferase
activity in intact rats. *Neuroscience Letters*, 1978a, *9*, 83.

Vaughan, G.M., McDonald, S.D., Jordan, R.M., Allen, J.P., Bell,
R., & Stevens, E.A. Melatonin, pituitary function and stress in
humans. *Psychoendocrinology*, 1979, *4*, 351.

Wetterberg, L. Melatonin in humans: physiological and clinical
studies. *Journal of Neural Transmission*, 1978, *13*, 289.

CHAPTER 12

Ader, R. Ed. *Psychoneuroimmunology*. New York, Academic Press,
1981.

Amkraut, A.A., Solomon, G.F., & Kraemer, H.C. Stress, early

experience and adjuvant-induced arthritis in the rat. *Psychosomatic Medicine*, 1971, *33*, 203.

Bonnys, M., & McKenzie, J.M. Interactions of stress and endocrine status on rat peripheral lymphocyte responsiveness to phytomitogens. *Psychoendocrinology*, 1978, *4*, 67.

Burchfield, S.R., Woods, S.C., & Mathews, S.E. Effects of cold stress on tumor growth. *Physiology & Behavior*, 1978, *21*, 537.

Elliot, E.V., & Sinclair, N.R. Effect of cortisone acetate on 19S and 7S haemolysin antibody. A time course study. *Immunology*, 1968, *15*, 643.

Eskola, J., Ruuskannen, O., Soppi, E., Viljanen, M., Jarvinen, M., Toivonen, H., & Kouvalainen, K. Effect of sport stress on lymphocyte transformation and antibody formation. *Clinical & Experimental Immunology*, 1978, *32*, 339.

Fabris, N., Pierpaoli, W., & Sorkin, E. In J. Sterzl & I. Riha, (Eds.) *Developmental Aspects of Antibody Formation and Structure*, (Vol. 1), Academic Publishing House of the Czecholslovak Academy of Sciences, Prague, 1970, *79*.

Gisler, R.H., & Schenkel-Hulliger, L. Hormonal regulation of the immune response. II. Influence of pituitary and adrenal activity on immune responsiveness. *Cellular Immunology*, 1971, *2*, 646.

Hadden, J.W., Hadden, E.M., & Middleton, Jr., E. Lymphocyte blast transformation. I. Demonstration of adrenergic receptors in human peripheral lymphocytes. *Cellular Immunology,* 1970, *1,* 583.

Joasoo, A., & McKenzie, J.M. Stress and immune response in rats. *International Archives of Allergy & Applied Immunology*, 1976, *50*, 659.

Johnson, T., Lavender, J.F., Hultin, E., & Rasmussen, Jr., A.F. The influence of avoidance-learning stress on resistance to Cocksackie B virus in mice. *Journal of Immunology*, 1963, *91*, 569.

MacManus, J.P., Whitfield, J.F., & Youdale, T. Stimulation by epinephrine of adenyl cyclase activity, cyclic AMP formation, DNA synthesis and cell proliferation in populations of rat lymphocytes. *Journal of Cellular & Comparative Physiology*, 1971, *77*, 103.

Monjan, A.A., & Collector, M.I. Stress-induced modulation of the immune response. *Science*, 1977, *196*, 307.

Newberry, B.H., Gildow, J., Wogan, J., & Reese, R.L. Inhibition of Huggins tumors by forced restraint. *Psychosomatic Medicine*, 1976, *38*, 155.

Nowell, P.C. Mitotic inhibition by epinephrine in leukocyte cultures. *Abstract. Proceedings of the Federation of American Societies of Experimental Biology*, 1962, *21*, 73.

Pavlidis, N., & Chirigos, M. Stress-induced impairment of macrophage tumoricidal function. *Psychosomatic Medicine*, 1980, *42*, 47.

Pierpaoli, W., Fabris, N., & Sorkin, E. In G.E. Wolstenholms & J. Knight (Eds.) *Hormones and the immune response*. London: Churchill, 1970.

Rashkis, H.A. Systematic stress as an inhibitor of experimental tumors in swiss mice. *Science*, 1952, *116*, 169.

Rasmussen, A.F., Jr., Emotions and immunity. *Annals of the New York Academy of Science*, 1969, *164*, 458.

Riley, V. Mouse mammary tumors: alteration of incidence as apparent function of stress. *Science*, 1975, *189*, 465.

Riley, V. Psychoneuroendocrine influences on immunocompetence and neoplasia. *Science*, 1981, *212*, 1100.

Sklar, L.S., & Anisman, H. Stress and coping factors influence tumor growth. *Science*, 1979, *205*, 513.

Sklar, L.S., & Anisman, H. Social stress influences tumor growth. *Psychosomatic Medicine*, 1980, *42*, 347.

Sklar, L.S., Bruto, V., & Anisman, H. Adaptation to the tumor-enhancing effects of stress. *Psychosomatic Medicine*, 1981, *43*, 331.

Solomon, G.F., & Moos, R.H. Emotions, immunity and disease: a speculative theoretical integration. *Archives of General Psychiatry*, 1964, *11*, 657.

Solomon, G.F. Stress and antibody response in rats. *Archives of Allergy and Applied Immunology*, 1969, *35*, 97.

Tobach, E., & Bloch, H. Effect of stress by crowding prior to and following tuberculosis infection. *American Journal of Physiology*, 1956, *187*, 399.

Udupa, K.N., Rao, A., Prasad, R., Khatri, S., Patel, V., & Chansouria, J.P.N. Role of stress in cancer. *Indian Journal of Cancer*, 1980, *17*, 7.

Wick, M.M. L-dopa methyl ester: prolongation of survival of

neuroblastoma-bearing mice after treatment. *Science*, 1978, *199*, 775.

Wick, M.M. L-dopa methyl ester as a new antitumor agent. *Nature*, 1977, *269*, 512.

Zimel, H., Zimel, A., Petrescu, R., Ghinea, E., & Tasca, C. Influence of stress and of endocrine imbalance on the experimental metastasis. *Neoplasma*, 1977, *24*, 151.

CHAPTER 13

Abrams, A., Braff, D., Janowsky, D., Hall, S., & Segal, D. Unresponsiveness of catatonic symptoms to naloxone. *Pharmakopsychiatry*, 1978, *11*, 177.

Akil, H., Madden, J., Patrick, R.L., & Barchas, J.D. In H.W. Kosterlitz (Ed.) *Opiates and endogenous opioid peptides*, Amsterdam: Elsevier, 1976.

Amir, S., Brown, Z.W., & Amit, Z. The role of endorphine in stress: evidence and speculations. *Neuroscience & Biobehavioral Reviews*, 1979, *4*, 77.

Amir, S., & Bernstein, M. Endogenous opioids interact in stress-induced hyperglycemia in mice. *Physiology and Behavior*, 1981, *28*, 575.

Änggard, E., & Jonsson, C.E., in P. W. Ramwell & B. B. Pharriss (eds.) *Prostaglandins in cellular biology*. New York: 1972.

Barchas, J.D., Akil, H. Elliot, G.R., Holman, R.B., & Watson, S.J. Behavior neurochemistry: neuroregulators and behavioral states. *Science*, 1978, *200*, 964.

Belenky, G.L., & Holaday, J.W. Repeated electroconvulsive shock (ECS) and morphine tolerance: demonstration of cross-sensitivity in the rat. *Life Sciences,* 1981, *29,* 553.

Bergström, S., Carlson, A., & Weeks, J.R. the prostaglandins: A family of biologically active lipids. *Pharmacological Reviews*, 1968, *20*, 1.

Blair, M.L., Feigl, E.O., & Smith, O.A. Elevation of plasma renin activity during avoidance performance in baboons. *American Journal of Physiology*, 1976, *231*, 772.

Cohen, M., Pickar, D., Dubois, M., Roth, Y.F., Naber, D., &

Bunney, W.E., Jr., Surgical stress and endorphins. *Lancet*, 1981, 213.

deWied, D., Witter, A., Versteeg, D.H.G., & Mulder, A.H. Release of ACTH by substances of central nervous system origin. *Endocrinology*, 1969, *85*, 561.

Ferriera, S.H., Flower, R., Moncada, S., & Vane, J.R. In G. Katona & J. R. Blengio (Eds.) *Inflammation and anti-inflammatory therapy*, New York: 1975.

Flack, J.D., Jessup, D.R., & Ramwell, P.W. Prostaglandin stimulation of rat corticosteroidogenesis. *Science*, 1969, *163*, 691.

Grandison, L., & Guidotti, A. Regulation of prolactin release by endogenous opiates. *Nature*, 1977, *270*, 357.

Gréen, K., & Samuelsson, B. Quantitative studies on the synthesis in vivo of prostaglandins in the rat. *European Journal of Biochemistry*, 1971, *22*, 391.

Guillemin, R., Vargo, T.M., Rossier, J., Minick, S., Ling, N., Rivier, C., Vale, W., & Bloom, F. B-endorphin and adrenocortico-tropin are secreted concomitantly by the pituitary gland, 1977, *197,* 1367.

Hanukoglu, I. Prostaglandins as first mediators of stress? *Lancet*, 1977, *I*, 193.

Hanukoglu, I. Prostaglandins as first mediators of stress. (letter) *New England Journal of Medicine*, 1977, 1414.

Harms, P.G., Langlier, P., & McCann, S.M. Modification of stress-induced prolactin release by dexamethasone or adrenalectomy. *Endocrinology,* 1975, *96,* 475.

Hayes, R.L., Bennett, G.J., Newlon, P.G., & Mayer, D.J. Behavioral and physiological studies of non-narcotic analgesia in the rat elicited by certain environmental stimuli. *Brain Research*, 1978, *155*, 69.

Hedge, G.A., & Hanson, S.D. The effects of prostaglandins on ACTH secretion. *Endocrinology*, 1972, *91*, 925.

Hedge, G.A. Hypothalamic and pituitary effects of prostaglandins on ACTH secretion. *Prostaglandins*, 1976, *11*, 293.

Horton, E.W. Hypotheses on physiological roles of prostaglandins. *Physiological Review*, 1969, *49*, 122.

Ipp, E., Dobbs, R., & Unger, R.H. Morphine and β-endorphin influence the secretion of the endocrine pancreas. *Nature*, 1978, *276*, 190.

Ipp, E., Schusdziarra, V., Harris, V., & Unger, R.H. Morphine-induced hyperglycemia. Role of insulin and glucagon. *Endocrinology*, 1980a, *107*, 461.

Ipp, E., Dhoranwala, J.W., Moossa, A.R., & Rubenstein, A.H. Enkephalin stimulates insulin and glucagon in vivo and accentuates hyperglycemia in diabetic dogs. *Clinical Research*, 1980b, *28*, 396A.

Januszewicz, W., Sznajderman, M., Wocial, B., Feltynowski, T., & Klonowicz, T. The effect of mental stress on catecholamines, their metabolites and plasma renin activity in patients with essential hypertension and in healthy subjects. *Clinical Science*, 1979, *57*, 229s.

Jindra, A., Jr., & Kvetnansky, R. Stress-induced activation of inactive renin. Molecular weight aspects. *Journal of Biological Chemistry*, 1982, *257*, 5997.

Kauter, R.A., Ensinck, J.W., & Fujimoto, W.Y. Desperate effects of enkephalin and morphine upon insulin and glucagon secretion by islet cell cultures. *Diabetes*, 1980, *29*, 84.

Kehlet, H., Brand, M., Enquist, A., & Madsen, S.N. Prostaglandins as mediators for stress, reaction. *New England Journal of Medicine*, 1977, *627*.

Kosterlitz, H.W. Endogenous opioid peptides and the control of pain. *Psychological Medicine*, 1979, *9*, 1.

Kosunen, K.J., Pakarinen, A.J., Kuoppasalmi, K., & Adlercreutz, H. Plasma renin activity, angiotensin II, and aldosterone during intense heat stress. *Journal of Applied Physiology*, 1976, *41*, 323.

Kountz, S.L. Acute effects of stress on renal function in healthy donors. *New York State Journal of Medicine*, 1975, *2138*.

Leenen, F.H., & Shapiro, A.P. Effect of intermittent electric shock on plasma renin activity in rats. *Proceedings of the Society of Experimental Biology & Medicine*, 1974, *146*, 534.

Lewis, J.W., Cannon, J.T., & Liebeskind, J.C. Opioid and nonopioid mechanisms of stress analgesia. *Science*, 1980, *208*, 623.

Lewis, J.W., Slater, S.J., Hall, J.L., Terman, G.W., & Liebeskind,

J.C. Chronic stress enhances morphine analgesia in the rat. *Proceedings of the Western Pharmacology Society*, 1982, *25*, 137.

Mains, R.E., Eipper, B.A., & Ling, M. Common precursor to corticotropins and endorphins. *Proceedings of the National Academy of Sciences*, USA, 1977, *74*, 3014.

Markelonis, G., & Garbus, J. Alterations in intracellular oxidative metabolism as stimuli evoking prostaglandin biosynthesis. *Prostaglandins*, 1975, *10*, 1087.

Markov, Kh.M., Bankova, V.V., & Kucherenko, A.G. Renin-angiotensin-aldosterone system in rats with neurogenic stress. *Byulleten 'Eksperimental 'noi Biologii i Meditsiny*, 1976, *82*, 1179.

North, R.A. Opiates, opioid peptides and single neurons. *Life Sciences*, 1979, *24*, 1527.

Peng, T.C., Six, K.M., & Munson, P.L. Effects of prostaglandin E_1 on the hypothalamo-hypophyseal-adrenocortical axis in rats. *Endocrinology*, 1970, *86*, 202.

Porte, D., & Robertson, R.P. Control of insulin secretion by catecholamines, stress and the sympathetic nervous system. *Federation Proceedings*, 1973, *32*, 1972.

Ramwell, P.W., & Shaw, J.E. Biological significance of the prostaglandins. *Recent Progress in Hormone Research*, 1970, *29*, 139.

Riley, A.L, Zellner, D.A., & Duncan, H.J. The role of endorphins in animal learning and behavior. *Neuroscience & Behavioral Reviews*, 1980, *4*, 69.

Rossier, J., French, E., Rivier, C., Ling, N., Guillemin, R., & Bloom, F.E. Foot shock induced stress increases β-endorphin levels in blood but not in brain. *Nature*, 1977, *270*, 618.

Rossier, J., French, E., Rivier, C., Shibasaki, T., Guillemin, R., & Bloom, F.E. Stress-induced release of prolactin: blockade by dexamethasone and naloxone may indicate β-endorphin mediation. *Proceedings National Academy of Sciences*, USA, 1980, *77*, 666.

Samuelsson, B., Granström, E., Green, K., Hamberg, M., & Hammarstrom, H. Prostaglandins. *Annual Review of Biochemistry*, 1975, *44*, 669.

Selye, H. *The physiology and pathology of exposure to stress*. Montreal Acta, 1950.

Selye, H. *The stress of life*. (2nd ed.). New York: McGraw-Hill, 1975.

Sherman, J.E., Lewis, J.W., deWetter, R.E., & Liebeskind, J.C. Conditioned fear enhances morphine analgesia in the rat. *Proceedings of the Western Pharmacological Society*, 1981, *24*, 327.

Sigg, E.B., Keim, K.L., & Sigg, T.D. On the mechanism of renin release by restraint stress in rats. *Pharmacology, Biochemistry & Behavior*, 1978, *8*, 47.

Syvalahti, E., Lammintausta, R., & Pekkarinen, A. Effect of psychic stress of examination on serum growth hormone, serum insulin, and plasma renin activity. *Acta Pharmacologica et Toxicologica*, 1976, *38*, 344.

Tannenbaum, G., Panerai, A.E., & Friesen, H.G. Failure of β-endorphin antiserum, naloxone and naltrexone to alter physiological growth hormone and insulin secretion. *Life Sciences*, 1983, *25*, 1979.

Tsukiyama, H., Otsuka, K., Kyuno, S., Fujishima, S., & Kijima, F. Influence of immobilization stress on blood pressure, plasma renin activity, and biosynthesis. *Japanese Circulation Journal*, 1973, *37*, 1265.

Vale, W., Rivier, C., & Guillemin, R. A "Prostaglandin Receptor" in the mechanisms involved in the secretion of anterior pituitary hormones. *Federation Proceedings*, 1971, *30*, 363.

Verebey, K., Volavka, J., & Clouet, D. Endorphins in psychiatry. *Archives of General Psychiatry*, Chicago, 1978, *35*, 877.

Wernze, H., Hilfenhaus, M., Rietbrock, I., Schüttke, R., & Kühn, K. Plasma-Renin-Activitat und Plasma-Aldosteron unter Narkose sowie Operationsstreß und Beta-Receptoren-Blockade. *Anaesthesie*, 1975 *24*, 471.

Wesche, D.L., & Frederickson, R.C.A. Diurnal differences in opioid peptide levels correlated with nociceptive sensitivity. *Life Sciences*, 1979, *24*, 1861.

Woods, S.C., & Porte, D. Neural control of the endocrine pancreas. *Physiological Review*, 1974, *54*, 596.

CHAPTER 14

Engleman, K., & Portnoy, B. A Sensitive double-isotope derivative assay for norepinephrine and epinephrine. Normal resting human plasma levels. *Circulation Research*, 1970, *26*, 53.

Goodman, L.S., & Gilman, A. *The pharmacological basis of therapeutics*, (6th ed.), New York: MacMillan Publishing Co., Inc. 1980.

Guyton, A.C. *Textbook of medical physiology*, (6th ed.) Philadelphia: W. B. Saunders Co., 1981.

Jacobson, E. Progressive relaxation. Chicago: University of Chicago Press, 1938.

Tepperman, J. Metabolic and endocrine physiology. Chicago: Year Book Medical Publishers, Inc., 1980.

Tietz, N.W. Fundamentals of clinical chemistry. Philadelphia: W. B. Saunders Co., 1976.

Williams, R.H. *Textbook of endocrinology*. Philadelphia: W. B. Saunders Co. 1981.

CHAPTER 15

Akiskal, H.S., and McKinney, W.T. Overview of recent research in depression. Integration of ten conceptual models into a comprehensive clinical frame. *Archives of General Psychiatry,* 1975, *32,* 285.

Cassel, J. Physical illness in response to stress. In S. Levine and N.A. Scotch (Eds.) *Social stress.* Chicago: Aldine Publishing Co., 1970.

Eliot, R. Stress and the major cardiovascular disorders. Mount Kisco, N.Y.: Futura, 1979.

Everly, G.S. Jr., & Rosenfeld, R. *The nature and treatment of the stress response.* New York: Plenum Press, 1981.

Fox, B.H. Premorbid psychological factors as related to cancer incidence. *Journal of Behaviorial Medicine,* 1978, *1,* 45.

Friedman, M. Pathogenesis of coronary artery disease. New York: McGraw-Hill, 1969.

Girdano, D.A., & Everly, G.S. *Controlling stress and tension: A holistic approach.* New Jersey: Prentice-Hall, Inc., 1979.

Glass, D.C. *Behavior patterns, stress, and coronary disease.* New Jersey: John Wiley & Sons, 1977.

Holmes, T.H., & Rahe, R.H. The social readjustment rating scale. *Journal of Psychosomatic Research.* 1967, *11,* 213.

Jenkins, C.D. Psychologic and social precursors of coronary disease. *New England Journal of Medicine,* 1971, *284,* 244.

Rosenman, R.H., Friedman, M., Straus, R., Jenkins, C.D., Zyzanski, S.J., & Wurm, M. Coronary heart disease in the western collaborative group study: a follow-up experience of 4½ years. *Journal of Chronic Diseases,* 1970, *23,* 173.

Selye, H. *The stress of life.* (2nd ed.) New York: McGraw-Hill Book Co., 1956, 1978.

Selye, H. *Stress in health and disease.* Reading, Mass: Butterworth's, 1976.

Straub, L.R., Ripley, H.S., & Wolf, S. Disturbances of bladder function associated with emotional stress. *Journal of American Medical Association,* 1949, *141,* 1139.

Weiss, J.J., Stone, E.A., & Harrell, N. Coping behavior and brain norepinephrine level in rats. *Journal of Comparative & Physiological Psychology,* 1970, *72,* 153.

Wilson, E.S., & Schneider, C. The neurophysiologic pathways of distress. *Stress/Pain Manager Newsletter,* S/P Management Group, Kansas City, Mo., May—Aug. 1981.

Wolff, H.G., Stress and disease. American Lecture Series, no. 166 Monograph in Bannerstone, Div. of American Lectures in Physiology. Springfield Illinois: Charles C. Thomas, 1953.

GLOSSARY

acetylcholine — A neurotransmitter substance secreted at the axon endings of many neurons that transmits an impulse across a synapse.

acoustic — Pertaining to the sense of hearing or sound.

acromegaly — Chronic disease characterized by elongation and enlargement of bones, of the extremities and certain head bones, especially frontal bone and jaws; accompanied by enlargement of nose and lips and thickening of soft tissues of the face.

action potential — The momentary difference in electrical potential between the active and resting sites of a nerve fiber; measured when the two sites are connected with a sensitive voltmeter.

adenine — One of the purine bases found in the nucleotides that constitute the subunits of DNA and RNA.

adenosine diphosphate (ADP) — The two-phosphate product of ATP breakdown; formed when ATP releases its stored energy. ATP → ADP + Pi + Energy.

adenosine monophosphate (AMP) — A monophosphate derivative of ATP; one of the nucleotides in DNA and RNA.

adenosine triphosphate (ATP) — Major energy carrier that transfers chemical potential energy from one molecule to another.

adenyl cyclase — Enzyme that catalyzes the transformation of ATP to cyclic AMP.

ADP — See adenosine diphosphate.

adrenal cortex — The outer layer of the adrenal gland which secretes mainly cortisol, aldosterone, and androgens.

adrenalectomy — Excision of the adrenal gland.

adrenal glands — Also called suprarenal glands; pair of endocrine glands located just above each kidney; each gland consists of two regions: an outer layer called the adrenal cortex and an inner core, called the adrenal medulla.

adrenaline — See epinephrine.

adrenal medulla — Inner portion of the adrenal gland which secretes both epinephrine and norepinephrine, but mainly epinephrine.

adrenergic fiber — Nerve fiber that secretes norepinephrine at the terminal end of its axon.

adrenocorticotropic hormone (ACTH) — Polypeptide hormone secreted by the anterior pituitary; stimulates some of the cells of the adrenal cortex; also called adrenocorticotropin, corticotropin.

afferent — Carrying impulses toward a center, as afferent sensory nerves carry messages toward the brain; also said of certain veins and lymphatics; opposite to efferent.

aldosterone — Mineralcorticoid steroid hormone secreted by the adrenal cortex; regulates electrolyte balance.

allergen — Foreign substance capable of stimulating an allergic reaction.

alpha adrenergic receptor — Type of receptor for norepinephrine and epinephrine that responds to certain drugs and can be distinguished from a beta-adrenergic receptor.

alveolus — Air sac of a lung, or other saclike structure; (plural: alveoli).

amenorrhea — Absence or suppression of menstruation; normal before puberty, after menopause, during pregnancy, and lactation.

amine — Type of nitrogen-containing organic compound, which includes the hormones secreted by the adrenal medulla.

amino acid — Organic compound of relatively small molecular size that contains an amino group ($-NH_2$) and a carboxyl group ($-COOH$); the structural unit of a protein molecule.

amniotic fluid — Fluid within the amniotic cavity that surrounds the developing fetus.

AMP — See adenosine monophosphate.

amygdala — Mass of gray matter in the anterior portion of the temporal lobe of the brain.

anabolism — Synthetic chemical reaction; reactions in which small molecular fragments come together to form larger molecules.

analgesia — Absence of normal sense of pain.

analgesic — Drug that relieves pain.

androgen — Male sex hormone such as testosterone.

angina — Any disease characterized by attacks of choking or suffocation; generally referred to some lesion of the coronary arteries of the heart, its valves or walls.

angiotensin I — Small polypeptide (10 amino acid residues) hormone generated in the blood by the action of renin on a plasma protein, angiotensinogen.

angiotensin II — Octapeptide formed by enzymatic removal of two amino acids from angiotensin I; stimulates the secretion of aldosterone from the adrenal cortex and the contraction of vascular smooth muscle.

angiotensin III — Heptapeptide formed by the enzymatic removal of an amino acid from angiotensin II.

angiotensinogen — Plasma protein synthesized in the liver; the precursor of the hormone angiotensin.

anterior pituitary — Anterior portion of the pituitary gland; synthesizes, stores and releases ACTH, GH, TSH, prolactin, FSH and LH.

antibody — Specialized protein secreted by plasma cells and capable of combining with the specific antigen that stimulated its production.

antidiuresis—Decrease in urine formation.

antidiuretic hormone (ADH)—Peptide hormone synthesized in the hypothalamus and released from the posterior lobe of the pituitary gland; it enhances the conservation of water by the kidneys; also known as vasopressin.

antigen — Substance which stimulates cells to produce antibodies.

apocrine glands — Type of sweat gland that responds during periods of emotional stress.

argenine vasopressin (AVP) — Substance which promotes antidiuresis.

arousal — When considered from a physiological point of view, pertains to the activation of the sympathetic portion of the autonomic nervous system.

arrhythmia — Abnormal heart activity characterized by a loss of rhythm.

arteriole — Small branch of an artery that communicates with the capillary network.

artery — Vessel that transports blood away from the heart.

assay — Analysis of a substance to determine its constituents and the relative proportion of each; physical, chemical, and biological methods are used.

ATP — See adenosine triphosphate.

atrium — Chamber of the heart that receives blood from the veins; (plural: atria).

atrophy — Wasting away or decrease in size of an organ or tissue.

autogenic training — Method that focuses on training the mind and body to respond quickly and effectively to verbal commands to relax and return to a balanced state.

autoimmune disease — Disease produced by antibodies or T cells sensitized against the body's own cells, which results in damage or alteration of cell function.

autonomic nervous system — Component of the efferent division of the peripheral nervous system; innervates cardiac muscle, smooth muscle, and glands; consists of sympathetic and parasympathetic subdivisions.

axon — That part of a neuron that conducts impulses away from the neuron cell body.

basal metabolic rate — Rate at which metabolic reactions occur when the body is at rest.

beta-adrenergic receptor — Type of receptor for norepinephrine and epinephrine that responds to certain drugs and can be distinguished from an alpha-adrenergic receptor.

beta cells — Basophilic cells in the anterior lobe of the hypophysis which give a positive periodic acid stain reaction. Cells of the islets of Langerhans of the pancreas which secrete insulin.

bioassay — Estimation of strength of a drug by noting its effect in a test animal and comparing such effects with a standard preparation.

biofeedback — A method or device used to feed back information on one's own physiological processes.

B-lymphocyte — lymphocyte that reacts against foreign substances in the body by producing and secreting antibodies.

bone marrow — Highly vascular, cellular substance in the central cavity of some bones; site of the synthesis of erythrocytes, some types of leukocytes, and platelets.

brainstem — Portion of the brain that includes the midbrain, pons, medulla oblongata, and diencephalon.

bronchiole — A small branch of a bronchus within the lung.

bronchoconstriction — Constriction of the lumen of the bronchi of the lungs.

bronchospasm — Spasm of the bronchus.

bronchus — A branch of the trachea that leads to a lung.

calcitonin — Hormone secreted by the thyroid gland that helps to regulate the level of blood calcium.

calorigenic — Pertaining to heat production or its increase.

cAMP — See cyclic AMP.

capillary — Small blood vessel that connects an arteriole and a venule.

cardiac output — Quantity calculated by multiplying the stroke volume by the heart rate.

cardiovascular system — Pertaining to the heart and blood vessels.

carotid — Pertaining to the two major arteries (the carotid arteries) in the neck that convey blood to the head.

carotid sinus — A small region in which there is a dilation of the internal carotid artery.

catabolism — Degradative chemical reactions that result in the fragmentation of molecules into smaller units.

catatonia — Phase of schizophrenia in which the patient is unresponsive; the tendency to assume and remain in a fixed posture, refusal to move or talk are characteristic of this phase.

catecholamine — Type of organic compound that includes epinephrine and norepinephrine.

cell membrane — Structural barrier composed of phospholipids and proteins associated with the cell surface and its organelles which provides a selective barrier to the movement of molecules and ions across the membrane; also see plasma membrane.

cellular physiology — Science of the function of cells, tissues, and organs of the living organism.

central nervous system (CNS) — Portion of the nervous system that consists of the brain and spinal cord.

cerebellum — Portion of the brain that coordinates skeletal muscle movements.

cerebral cortex — 3mm-thick cellular layer that covers the cerebrum.

cerebrum — Portion of the brain that occupies the upper part of the cranial cavity.

cesarean section — Removal of the fetus by means of an incision into the uterus, usually by way of the abdominal wall.

cGMP — See cyclic GMP.

cholesterol — Lipid produced by the cells of the body that is used in the synthesis of steroid hormones and is excreted into the bile.

cholinergic fiber — Nerve fiber that secretes acetylcholine at the terminal end of its axon.

chronotropic — Refers to any substance that affects the heart rate.

circadian rhythm — Pattern of repeated behavior associated with the cycles of night and day.

CNS — See central nervous system.

coagulation — Refers to the clotting of blood.

congenital — Condition present at the time of birth.

corpus luteum — Ovarian structure formed from the follicle after ovulation; secretes estrogen and progesterone.

cortex — Outer layer of an organ such as the adrenal gland, cerebrum, or kidney.

cortical — Pertaining to the cortex.

cortical fibers — Fibers of the cortex.

corticoid — Anyone of a number of steroid substances obtained from the cortex of the adrenal gland; also called corticosteroid, glucocorticoids.

corticosteroid — See corticoid.

corticosterone — Hormone secreted by the adrenal cortex which influences carbohydrate metabolism; it is essential for normal absorption of glucose, the formation of glycogen in the liver and tissues and the normal utilization of carbohydrates by the tissues.

corticotropin — See adrenocorticotropin.

corticotropin releasing hormone (CRH) — Hypothalamic hormone that stimulates ACTH (corticotropin) secretion by the anterior pituitary.

cortisol — Glucocorticoid secreted by the adrenal cortex. It is the main glucocorticoid in humans.

craniosacral division — See parasympathetic nervous system.

cranium — Bones of the skull that enclose and protect the brain.

cyclic AMP (cAMP) — Cyclic 3', 5' — adenosine monophosphate, a cyclic nucleotide that serves as second messenger for many nonsteroid hormones, neurotransmitters, and paracrine agents.

cyclic GMP (cGMP) — cyclic 3', 5' — Guanosine monophosphate; a cyclic nucleotide that acts as second messenger in some cells, possibly in opposition to cyclic AMP.

cyclic guanosine monophosphate — See cyclic GMP.

cytoplasm — Contents of a cell surrounding its nucleus.

cytosol — Watery medium inside cells but outside of cell organelles.

dendrite — Branched cytoplasmic process of a neuron which conducts impulses to the cell body. There are usually several to a neuron and form synaptic connections with other neurons.

deoxyribonucleic acid (DNA) — Nucleic acid that stores and transmits genetic information; consists of a double strand (double helix) of nucleotide subunits; the sequence of nucleotides in DNA (three nucleotides specify one amino acid) determines the sequence of amino acids in the proteins.

depolarization — The process of changing the electrical potential across a muscle or nerve cell in a less negative direction.

diabetes mellitus — Condition characterized by a high blood glucose level and the appearance of glucose in the urine due to a deficiency of insulin.

diabetogenic agent — Any agent that causes the condition of diabetes.

diastolic pressure — The pressure measured in the arteries at the time of the greatest cardiac relaxation.

diencephalon — Portion of the brain in the region of the third ventricle that includes the thalamus and hypothalamus.

diuresis — Large or abnormal secretion of urine.

diuretic — Substance that causes an increased production of urine.

diurnal — Daily; occurring in a 24-hr. cycle.

DNA — See deoxyribonucleic acid.

dopamine — Catecholamine neurotransmitter; a precursor of epinephrine and norepinephrine.

dwarf — Abnormally short or undersized person.

effector organ — Organ such as a muscle or a gland that responds to stimulation.

efferent — Carrying away from, as efferent nerves which conduct impulses from the brain or spinal cord to the periphery, efferent lymph vessels which convey lymph from lymph nodes, and efferent arterioles which carry blood away from the glomeruli of the kidney.

electrocardiography — The making and study of graphic records (electrocardiograms—EKG) produced by electrical currents originating in the heart.

electrodermal measurement — Measurement of the electrical characteristics of the skin such as conductance, resistance or skin potential measurements.

electroencephalography — The recording and study of graphic records (electroencephalogram — EEG) produced by electrical fluctuations of the brain after amplification of more than a billion times.

electrolyte — Substance that ionizes in solution. The important ions in the body include Na⁺, K⁺, Cl⁻, and HCO₃⁻.

electromyography — Study of and interpretation of electromyograms (EMG) which are graphic displays of muscle contractions as a result of electrical stimulation.

electrophysiological — Branch of physiology which deals with the relationship of body processes to electrical phenomena such as the effects of electrical stimulation upon cells and tissues, and the production of electrical impulses by cells, tissues and organs.

endocrine gland — Gland that secretes hormones directly into the blood stream.

endogenous — Produced within a cell or organism.

endogenous morphines — See endogenous opiates.

endogenous opiates — Opiates produced within a cell or organism, e.g, endorphins; also called endogenous morphines.

end-organ — Expanded end of a nerve fiber in a peripheral structure; encapsulated termination of a nerve fiber which serves as a receptor; also refers to an actual organ or system in the body which may manifest dysfunction as a result of chronic stress reactivity.

endorphins—Group of peptides; some are probably neurotransmitters at the synapses activated by opiate drugs; also called endogenous morphines or endogenous opiates.

enkephalin — Peptide that possibly functions as a neurotransmitter at the synapses activated by opiate drugs.

enzyme — Protein that is synthesized by a cell and acts as a catalyst in a specific cellular reaction.

eosinophil — White blood cell characterized by the presence of cytoplasmic granules that become stained by the acidic dye eosin.

epigastric region — Upper middle portion of the abdomen.

epinephrine — Hormone secreted by the adrenal medulla and involved in the regulation of metabolism, a catecholamine neurotransmitter; also called adrenaline.

epiphysis — See pineal gland.

estrogen — Hormone that stimulates the development of female secondary sex characteristics.

etiology — Study of the causes of disease which result from an abnormal state producing pathological conditions.

exocrine gland — Gland that secretes its products into a duct or onto a body surface.

exogenous — Originating outside an organ or part.

extrahypothalamic — Outside the hypothalamus.

fatty acid — Organic substance that serves as a building block for a fat molecule.

feedback — Situation in which the ultimate effects of a system influences the system itself; see also negative feedback, positive feedback.

fetus — Human embryo after eight weeks of development.

fibroblast — Cell that functions to produce fibers and other intercellular materials in connective tissues.

"fight or flight" response — Activation of the sympathetic adrenal medullary axis.

first messenger — Pertaining to the initial stimulating hormone.

follicle stimulating hormone (FSH) — Polypeptide hormone secreted by the anterior pituitary in both males and females; one of the gonadotropins which act on the gonads.

follicular cell — Cell of the ovarian follicle.

frontal cortex — Anterior cortex.

frontalis muscle — Portion of the occipito-frontalis muscle which covers the whole of one side of the vertex of the skull, from the occiput to the eyebrow.

galvanic skin response (GSR) — Electrical characteristics of the skin (see electrodermal measurements).

ganglion — Mass of neuron cell bodies usually outside the central nervous system.

gastrointestinal system — Gastrointestinal tract plus the salivary glands, portion of the liver and the pancreas; pertaining to the stomach and intestine.

gastrointestinal tract — Mouth, esophagus, stomach, small and large intestines.

general adaptation syndrome (GAS) — Theoretical concept used to describe the series of nervous and endocrine gland activities that take place during the chronic phase of stress reactivity; GAS is characterized by three stages, the alarm reaction, the stage of resistance and the stage of exhaustion.

gestation — Period of intrauterine fetal development also known as fetation; gravidity; pregnancy.

giantism — Abnormal development of the body or its parts.

glucagon — Hormone secreted by the pancreatic islets of Langerhans that causes the release of glucose from stored glycogen.

glucocorticoid — Anyone of a group of hormones secreted by the adrenal cortex that influence carbohydrate, fat, and protein metabolism.

glucogenolysis — Breakdown of glycogen.

gluconeogenesis — Formation of glucose from noncarbohydrate sources such as proteins and possibly fats; it occurs in the liver under such conditions as low carbohydrate intake or starvation.

glucose — Monosaccharide found in blood that serves as the primary source of cellular energy.

glutamic acid — Amino acid that is formed during the hydrolysis of proteins.

glycine — Amino acid derived from gelatin and from many proteins.

glycogenolysis — Conversion of glycogen into dextrose in the liver.

gonad — Reproductive organ; an ovary or testis.

gonadectomy — Excision of a testis or ovary.

gonadotropin-releasing hormone (GnRH) — Hypothalamic hormone that controls LH & FSH secretion by the anterior pituitary.

granulosa cells — Cells that line the antrum in the ovarian follicle.

growth — Increase in body size; i.e., lengthening of the long bones, increased cell division and cell volume, and accumulation of protein.

growth hormone (GH) — Hormone released by the anterior lobe of the pituitary gland that promotes the growth of the organism. Also called somatotropin or somatotropic hormone (STH).

growth hormone inhibiting hormone (GHIH) — See somatostatin.

growth hormone releasing hormone (GHRH) — Hypothalamic hormone that stimulates the secretion of growth hormone (GH) by the anterior pituitary.

GSR — See galvanic skin response.

guanine — One of the purine bases in DNA & RNA.

halothane — Fluorinated hydrocarbon used as a general anesthetic.

HCG — See human chorionic gonadotropin.

hemoconcentration — Increase in the number of red blood cells resulting from a decrease in the volume of plasma.

hemodynamics — Study of the circulation of the blood.

heparin — Substance that interferes with the formation of a blood clot; an anticoagulant.

hepatic — Pertaining to the liver.

hippocampus — Elevation of the floor of the inferior horn of the lateral ventricle of the brain, occupying nearly all of it.

homeostasis — Refers to an equilibrium state in which the internal physical and chemical environment of the body stays relatively constant.

homeostatic cybernetic control — Control system that consists of a collection of interconnected components and functions to keep a physical or chemical parameter of the internal environment relatively constant.

hormone — Substance secreted by an endocrine gland that is transmitted directly into the blood.

human chorionic gonadotropin (HCG) — Hormone produced by the placenta during pregnancy.

17-hydroxycorticosteroid (17-OHCS). Metabolic endproducts of cortisol metabolism.

5-hydroxytryptamine — See serotonin.

hyperglycemia — Excessively high level of blood glucose.

hyperphosphatemia — Abnormal amount of phosphorus in the blood; also called hyperphospheremia.

hyperthermia — Usually high fever.

hyperventilation — Overventilation; increase in the inspiration and expiration of air due to an increase in the rate or depth of respiration or both; results in carbon dioxide decrease below normal with possible resulting symptoms such as a decrease in blood pressure, vasoconstriction, and syncope.

hypoadrenalism — Adrenal insufficiency; also known as hypoadrenia.

hypocalcemia — Abnormally low blood calcium.

hypoglycemia — Deficiency of sugar in the blood. A condition in which there is less than 80 mg of sugar per 100cc of blood.

hypokinesia — Decreased motor reaction to a stimulus.

hypophyseal stalk — Means by which the hypophysis is attached to the hypothalamus; also known as pituitary stalk.

hypophysis — See pituitary gland.

hypothalamic releasing factors — See hypothalamic releasing hormones.

hypothalamic releasing hormones — Hormones released from hypothalamic neurons into the hypothalamopituitary portal vessels to control the release of the anterior pituitary hormones; formerly called hypothalamic releasing factors.

hypothalamus — Portion of the brain located below the thalamus, forming the floor of the third ventricle.

hypothermia — Having a body temperature below normal.

hypothyroidism — Low secretion of thyroid hormones.

Hz — Hertz — A unit to measure wave patterns in cycles per second.

immunity — Resistance to the effects produced by specific disease causing agents.

immunology — Study of immunity to diseases.

initial segment — Initial or beginning segment of the axon.

insulin — Hormone secreted by the islets of Langerhans that functions in the control of carbohydrate metabolism.

intercellular — Between cells.

intercellular fluid — Tissue fluid located between cells, other than blood cells.

interoceptive — Pertaining to taste.

interstitial cell stimulating hormone (ICSH) — See luteinizing hormone.

ionotropic — Refers to any substance that affects the force of contraction of the heart.

islands of Langerhans — The clusters of endocrine cells in the pancreas that produce insulin, glucagon, and somatostatin; also known as islets of Langerhans.

kidney — One of two glandular, bean shaped bodies, purplish-brown in color, situated at the back of the abdominal cavity, one on each side of the spinal column, which excrete waste products from the body in the form of urine.

lacrimal gland — Tear secreting gland.

lactation — Production of milk by the mammary glands.

larynx — Structure located between the pharynx and trachea that houses the vocal cords.

leukemia—Disease of unknown cause characterized by rapid and abnormal proliferation of leukocytes in the blood forming organs, and in the presence of immature leukocytes in the peripheral circulation; may be acute or chronic, but generally fatal.

leukocytes—Refers to the different types of white blood cells; also written as leucocytes.

limbic system—Group of interconnected structures within the brain that functions to produce various emotional feelings.

lipolysis — Decomposition or breakdown of fat.

lumbar — Pertaining to the region of the loins.

luteinizing hormone (LH) — Polypeptide secreted by the anterior pituitary which acts upon the gonads; one of the gonadotropins; sometimes called interstitial cell-stimulating hormone (ICSH) in the male.

luteinizing hormone releasing hormone (LHRH) — See gonadotropin-releasing hormone (GnRH), (GRH).

lymph — Fluid transported by the lymphatic vessels.

lymph node — Mass of lymphoid tissue located along the course of a lymphatic vessel.

lymphocyte — Type of white blood cell produced in lymphatic tissue.

lymphoid tissue — Lymph nodes, spleen, thymus, tonsils, and aggregates of lymphoid follicles such as those that line the gastrointestinal tract.

lymphoma — Lymphoid tissue tumor.

lysosome — Cytoplasmic organelle that contains digestive enzymes.

macula densa — A specialized group of cells in the kidney responsible for the production of renin.

mammary glands — Milk-secreting glands in the breasts.

meconium — First feces of a newborn infant composed of salts, mucus, bile and epithelial cells; almost odorless and of tarry consistency; evacuated by the third or fourth day after birth.

medulla — Inner portion of an organ such as the adrenal gland, cerebrum, or kidney.

medulla oblongata — Portion of the brain stem located between the pons and the spinal cord.

melanin — Pigment which gives color to hair, skin, and the choroid of the eye, and is present in some cancers, as in Melanoma.

melanocyte stimulating hormone (MSH) — Hormone secreted by the pars intermedia of the pituitary gland.

melanogenesis — Formation of melanin, or melanin production.

melanophore — Cell carrying dark pigment.

melatonin — Hormone thought to be secreted by the pineal gland.

membrane permeability — Ability of a membrane to permit the passage of water and certain substances in solution.

menstrual cycle — Cyclic rise and fall in female reproductive hormones; a period approximately 28 days in female human beings.

mesencephalic or mesencephalon — Midbrain consisting of the corpora quadrigemina, the crura cerebri, and the aqueduct of Sylvius.

metabolism — All the chemical reactions that occur within a living organism.

metabolite — Any product of metabolism.

microorganism — Minute living body not perceptible to the naked eye, especially a bacterium, protozoon, or virus.

midbrain — Small region of the brainstem located between the diencephalon and the pons.

mineralocorticoid — any one of a group of hormones secreted by the adrenal cortex that influences the concentrations of electrolytes in body fluids.

monocyte — Type of white blood cell that functions as a phagocyte.

morphine — Main alkaloid found in opium, occurring in bitter, colorless crystals; widely used as an analgesic and sedative.

MSHIH — Hypothalamic hormone that inhibits the secretion of MSH from the pituitary.

mucosa — Membrane that lines tubes and body cavities that open to the outside of the body.

muscarinic receptor — Acetylcholine receptors that can be stimulated by the mushroom poison muscarine; most of these receptors are on smooth muscles and gland cells.

myocardial contractility — Contractility of the myocardium.

myocardium — Muscle tissue of the heart.

myoepithelial cells — Specialized contractile cells that surround the alveoli of mammary glands.

negative feedback — Aspect of systems in which the ultimate effects of the system counteract the original stimulus.

neocortex or neocortical level — Portion of cerebral hemisphere not belonging to the rhinencephalon or corpus striatum, comprising most of the convoluted cortex and its associated white fibers.

neonatal — Pertaining to the period of life from birth to the end of four weeks.

neoplastic — Pertaining to, or of the nature of new, abnormal tissue formation.

nephron — Functional unit of the kidney.

neuroendocrinology — The study of the interrelationships between the nervous and the endocrine systems.

neurogenic — Originating from the nervous tissue; due to or resulting from nervous impulses.

neurohumor — Hormone; a chemical substance liberated at a nerve-ending which excites or activates an adjacent structure (neuron or muscle fiber).

neurohypophysis — Posterior lobe of the pituitary gland.

neuromodulator — Chemical that amplifies or dampens neuronal activity by altering the neurons directly or by influencing the effectiveness of a neurotransmitter; does not act as a specific neurotransmitter.

neuron — Nerve cell that consists of a cell body, soma, axon, and its processes (dendrites). The structural and functional unit of the nervous system.

neurophysiology — Physiology of the nervous system of the body.

neurosis — Mental or psychic disorder irrespective of etiology. Minor disorders are called neuroses; major ones, psychoses.

neurotic — One suffering from the instability of the nervous system; nervous or pertaining to a neurosis.

neurotransmitter — Chemical substance released by one neuron that acts upon a second neuron or upon a muscle or gland cell that alters its electrical state or activity.

neurotrophic — Pertains to the influence of nervous impulses upon the well-being of an organ or structure.

neurotropic — See neurotrophic.

neutrophil — Type of phagocytic leukocyte.

nicotine — Poisonous alkaloid found in all parts of the tobacco plant but especially in the leaves.

nicotinic receptors — Acetylcholine receptors that respond to the drug nicotine; primarily, the receptors at the motor end plate and the receptors on postganglionic neurons of the autonomic nervous system.

noradrenaline — See norepinephrine.

norepinephrine (noradrenaline) — Hormone produced by the adrenal medulla similar in chemical and pharmacologic properties to epinephrine but differing in possessing an N-methyl group.

nuclear protein — Protein portion of chromatin; involved in the control of gene activity.

nucleic acid — Substance composed of nucleotides bonded together; DNA or RNA.

nucleotide — Molecular subunit of nucleic acids that consist of a purine or pyrimidine base, a sugar, and phosphoric acid.

nucleus — Body within a cell that contains relatively large quantities of DNA; or the dense core of an atom which is composed of protons and neutrons.

17-OHCS — See 17-hyrdoxycorticosteroids.

olfactory — Pertaining to the sense of smell.

opiate — Drug derived from opium that induces sleep.

optic — Pertaining to the eye.

optic chiasma — X-shaped structure on the underside of the brain created by a partial crossing-over of fibers in the optic nerves.

organelle — Living part of a cell that performs a specialized function.

organism — Living thing, plant or animal. May be unicellular (bacteria, yeasts, protozoa) or multicellular (all complex organisms including humans.)

osmoreceptor — Receptor that is sensitive to changes in the osmotic pressure of body fluids.

osmosis — Diffusion of water through a selectively permeable membrane due to the presence of a concentration gradient across the membrane.

osmotic pressure — Pressure which develops when two solutions of different concentrations are separated by a semipermeable membrane.

osteoclasts — Cells that cause the erosion of bone.

ovarian follicle — Ovum and its encasing follicular, granulosa, and theca cells at any stage of its development prior to ovulation.

ovary — Primary reproductive organ of a female; an egg-cell-producing organ.

ovulation — Release of an ovum from the ovary.

ovum — Female gamete that is fertilized by a sperm cell at the time of conception; (plural: ova).

oxytocin — Hormone released by the posterior lobe of the pituitary gland that causes contraction of smooth muscles in the uterus and mammary glands.

pancreas — Glandular organ in the abdominal cavity that secretes hormones and digestive enzymes.

paracrine — Referring to the release of locally acting substances from endocrine cells.

parasympathetic nervous system — Portion of the autonomic nervous system that arises from the cranial and sacral region of the spinal cord.

parathormone — See parathyroid hormone (PTH).

parathyroid — Four small endocrine glands that are embedded in the posterior portion of the thyroid gland which secrete parathyroid hormone (PTH).

parathyroid hormone (PTH) — Peptide hormone secreted by the parathyroid glands; also called parathormone; regulates calcium and phosphate concentrations in the body.

paroxysm — Sudden periodic attack or recurrence of symptoms of a disease; an exacerbation of the symptoms of a disease.

pars distalis — Part of the hypophysis forming the major portion of the anterior lobe.

pars intermedia — Intermediate lobe of the hypophysis.

pathophysiology — Branch of physiology dealing with the process of disease.

peptide — Short polypeptide chain.

peripheral — Pertaining to parts located near the surface or toward the outside.

peripheral nervous system (PNS) — Portions of the nervous system outside the central nervous system.

peristalsis — Rhythmic waves of muscular contractions that occur in the walls of various tubular organs such as the intestine.

permeable membrane — See membrane permeability.

phagocyte — Cell which has the ability to engulf and digest solid substances.

pharynx — Portion of the digestive tract between the mouth and the esophagus.

pheocromocytoma — Tumor produced by the hypersecretion of epinephrine and norepinephrine; usually occurs in the adrenal medulla and is generally benign.

phospholipid — Lipid that contains phosphorus.

PIH — See prolactin inhibiting hormone.

pilo — Pertaining to hair.

pineal gland — Small structure located in the central part of the brain; also called epiphysis.

pituitary gland — Endocrine gland which is attached to the base of the brain, just below the hypothalamus. It consists of anterior, intermediary, and posterior lobes. Also called the hypophysis or hypophyseal gland.

plasma — Fluid, noncellular portion of the blood; a component of the extracellular fluid compartment.

plasma cells — Cells that are derived from lymphocytes and secrete antibodies.

plasma membrane — Cell membrane that forms the outer surface of the cell and separates its contents from the surrounding extracellular fluid; see cell membrane.

plethysmography — Measurement of variations in size of a part due to vascular changes; measurement of blood flow.

PNS — See peripheral nervous system.

polypeptide — Compound formed by the combination of many amino acid molecules.

pons — Portion of the brain stem above the medulla oblongata and below the midbrain.

positive chronotropic effect — Pertaining to an increase in the heartbeat.

positive feedback — Aspect of systems control in which the ultimate effects of the system influence it in such a way that these effects are increased, i.e., the original stimulus is strengthened.

positive inotropic effect — Pertaining to an increase in the force of contraction of the heart.

posterior pituitary — Portion of the pituitary from which oxytocin and antidiuretic hormone are released.

postganglionic fiber — Nerve fiber located on the distal side of a ganglion.

postsynaptic neuron — Neuron that conducts information away from a synapse, a neuron acted upon by a synapse.

precursor — Substance from which another substance is formed.

preganglionic fiber — Nerve fiber located on the proximal side of a ganglion.

presynaptic neuron — Neuron that conducts information toward a synapse.

PRH — See prolactin releasing hormone.

prolactin (P) — Hormone secreted by the anterior pituitary gland that stimulates the production of milk from the mammary glands.

prolactin inhibiting hormone (PIH) — hypothalamic hormone that inhibits prolactin secretion by the anterior pituitary.

prolactin releasing hormone (PRH) — Hypothalamic hormone that stimulates prolactin secretion by the anterior pituitary.

prostaglandins — Group of unsaturated modified fatty acids that function as chemical messengers; synthesized in most and possibly all cells of the body.

protein — Nitrogen-containing organic compound composed of amino acid molecules joined together.

psoriasis — Chronic inflammatory skin disease of many varieties characterized by formation of scaly red patches on exterior surfaces of the body.

psychogenic — Of mental origin.

psychophysiology — Science of the correlation of the physiological processes of the body and psychological processes of the mind and emotions.

psychosocial — Mental and/or emotional responses resulting from social interactions or lack of such interactions.

psychosomatic — Relating to or resulting from the interaction and interdependence of psychological somatic phenomena; of or relating to psychosomatics or psychosomatic disorders. One who evidences body symptoms or bodily and mental symptoms as a result of mental and/or emotional conflict.

pyloric sphincter — Ring of smooth muscle and connective tissue between the terminal antrum of the stomach and the first segment of the small intestine.

Raynaud's syndrome — Severe paroxysmal vascular disorder causing disturbances of the circulation in the extremities.
receptor — In sensory systems, it refers to the specialized peripheral
   ending of an afferent neuron or a separate cell intimately connected to it that detects changes in some aspect of the environment; in chemical communication, it refers to specific proteins either in the plasma membrane or cytosol of a target cell
   with which a chemical mediator combines to exert its effects.
releasing factors — See hypothalamic releasing hormones.
renal tubules — Portion of a nephron that extends from the renal
   corpuscle to the collecting duct.
ribonuclei acid (RNA) — Nucleic acid involved in the decoding of
   genetic information and its transfer to the site of protein synthesis; its nucleotides contain the sugar ribose to which is attached one of four bases (adenine, guanine, cytosine, or uracil);
   exists in three forms; messenger RNA, ribosomal RNA, and
   transfer RNA.
RNA — See ribonucleic acid.
repolarization — Reestablishment of the resting polarized state in a
   muscle or nerve fiber following conduction of a nerve impulse.
respiratory system — Structures involved in the exchange of gases
   between the blood and the external environment, i.e., the
   lungs, the diaphragm, and the series of airways that lead into
   the lungs; chest structures responsible for movement of air in
   and out of the lungs.
reticular formation — Complex network of nerve fibers within the
   brain stem that functions in arousing the cerebrum.

sacral — Pertaining to the sacrum.
sacrum — Triangular bone situated dorsal and caudal from the 2 ilia
   between the 5th lumbar vertebra and the coccyx.
saliva — Secretory product of the salivary glands; a watery solution
   of various salts and proteins.
second messenger — Pertaining to an intracellular hormone (e.g.
   cAMP), stimulated by an initial interacting hormone, and ini-
   tiates the intracellular physiological response characteristic of
   the initial hormone.

sensory nerve — Nerve composed of sensory nerve fibers.

septum — Membranous wall dividing two cavities.

serotonin (5-hydroxytryptamine, 5HT) — Probable neurotransmitter; vasoconstricting substance that is released by blood platelets when blood vessels are broken and thus helps to control bleeding.

sexual differentiation — Development of male or female reproductive organs.

sinus — Cavity or hollow space in a bone or other body part.

skin resistance — A measure of the reciprocal of skin conductivity and therefore a measure of sweat gland activity. This factor is increased during stress.

soma — Neuronal cell body or axon.

somatic nervous system — Component of the efferent division of the peripheral nervous system distinguished from the autonomic nervous system; innervates skeletal muscles.

somatostatin — Hypothalamic hormone that inhibits growth hormone and TSH secretion by the anterior pituitary; a possible neurotransmitter; found also in stomach and β cells of the pancreatic islets of Langerhans.

sphincter — Circular muscle that functions to close the lumen of a tubular structure.

spinal cord — Portion of the central nervous system extending downward from the brain stem through the vertebral canal.

splanchnic — Pertaining to the viscera.

spleen — Large glandular organ located in the upper left region of the abdomen.

steroid — Organic substance whose molecules include complex rings of carbon and hydrogen atoms.

stimulus — Change of environment of sufficient intensity to evoke a response in an organism.

stress management — Systematic program that is multidisciplinary in nature, which focuses on the mental, emotional and physical aspects of the human being in order to better cope with and manage the experience of stress in the human body.

stressor — Agent or condition capable of producing stress.

sympathetic nervous system — Portion of the autonomic nervous system whose preganglionic fibers leave the central nervous system at the thoracic and lumbar portions of the spinal cord.

sympathomimetic — Producing effects similar to those of the sympathetic nervous system.

synapse — Junction between the axon end of one neuron and the dendrite or cell body of another neuron.

synaptic cleft — Distance between two nerve terminals or one nerve terminal and a muscle cell, approximately 500 angstrom units.

syncope — Fainting or swooning. A transient form of unconsciousness, during which the person slumps to the ground resulting from cerebral anoxia.

systolic pressure — The pressure measured in the arteries during the greatest force exerted by the heart and the highest degree of resistance put forth by the arterial walls.

sweat glands — Simple coiled tubular glands found on most surfaces. The secreting portion lies in the subcutaneous portion of the skin. The excretory duct follows a winding course through the dermis and passes through the epidermis to its opening, a "sweat pore".

tactile — Pertaining to the touch.

target tissue — Specific tissue on which a hormone acts.

temporal lobe — Lobe of the cerebrum located laterally and below the frontal and occipital lobes. Contains auditory and receptive areas.

testis — Primary reproductive organ of the male; produces sperm cells.

thalamus — Mass of gray matter located at the base of the cerebrum in the wall of the third ventricle.

theca cells — Cell layer formed from follicle cells and specialized ovarian connective-tissue cells; surrounds the granulosa cells of the ovarian follicle.

thoracic — Pertaining to the chest.

thoracolumbar division — See sympathetic nervous system.

thymicolymphatic involution — Refers to the depression of immune activity along with the involution of the thymus gland.

thymosin — Hormone secreted by the thymus gland that has T lymphocytes as its target cells; thymic lymphopoietic factor.

thymus — Two-lobed glandular organ located in the mediastinum behind the sternum and between the lungs.

thyroidectomy — Removal of the thyroid gland.

thyroid gland — Endocrine gland located just below the larynx and in front of the trachea that secretes thyroid hormones.

thyroid-stimulating hormone (TSH) — Glycoprotein hormone secreted by the anterior pituitary; also called thyrotropin.

thyroid stimulating hormone releasing hormone — See thyrotropin-releasing hormone (TRH).

thyrotropin-releasing hormone (TRH) — Hypothalamic hormone that stimulates TSH (thyrotropin) secretion by the anterior pituitary.

thyroxine (T_4) — Iodine containing amino acid hormone secreted by the thyroid gland; also called tetraiodothyronine.

T-lymphocyte — Lymphocytes that interact directly with antigen-bearing particles and are responsible for cellular immunity.

toxin — Substance that is harmful to the body.

trachea — Tubular structure that leads from the larynx to the bronchi.

transcription — Formation of mRNA so that it contains in the linear sequence of its nucleotides the genetic information contained in the DNA gene from which of the mRNA is transcribed; the first stage in the transfer of information from DNA to protein synthesis.

trauma — Injury or wound.

triglyceride — Lipid composed of three fatty acids combined with a glycerol molecule.

triiodothyronine (T_3) — One of the thyroid hormones.

tropic hormone — Hormone that has an endocrine gland as its target tissue.

Type A personality — Personality type characterized by attitudes and behavior that lead to an elevated risk of coronary heart disease; this is in contrast to Type B personality which leads to little or no coronary risk.

umbilical cord — Cordlike structure that connects the fetus to the placenta.

urine — Fluid secreted from the blood by the kidneys stored in the bladder, and discharged, usually voluntarily by the urethra.

urticaria — Inflammation characterized by the eruption of pale, evanescent growths, accompanied by itching.

uterus — Hollow muscular organ located within the female pelvis in which the fetus develops.

vagina — Tubular organ that leads from the uterus to the vestibule of the female reproductive tract.

vagus nerve — Cranial nerve X; consists of approximately 90 percent afferent and 10 percent parasympathetic preganglionic efferent fibers. It is a nerve which has both motor and sensory functions and is more widely distributed than any of the other cranial nerves.

vascular — Pertaining to blood vessels.

vascular constriction — Constriction of blood vessels.

vascularization — Development of new blood vessels in a structure.

vasoconstriction — Decrease in the diameter of a blood vessel.

vasodilation — Increase in the diameter of a blood vessel.

vasomotor activity — Pertaining to the nerves having muscular control of the blood vessel wall.

vein — Vessel that carries blood toward the heart.

ventricle — Cavity such as those of the brain which are filled with cerebrospinal fluid or those of the heart which contain blood.

venule — Small thin-walled vessel that carries blood from a capillary network to a vein.

viscera — Organs in the thoracic and abdominal cavities.

weak phagocytes — White blood cells that engulf and digest solid substances.

zona fasciculata — Center zone of adrenal cortex.

zona glomerulosa — Outer zone of adrenal cortex.

zona reticularis — Inner zone of adrenal cortex.

INDEX